William Warfield

The Theory and Practice of Cattle-Breeding

William Warfield

The Theory and Practice of Cattle-Breeding

ISBN/EAN: 9783337143541

Printed in Europe, USA, Canada, Australia, Japan

Cover: Foto ©ninafisch / pixelio.de

More available books at **www.hansebooks.com**

THE THEORY AND PRACTICE

—OF—

CATTLE-BREEDING.

BY

WILLIAM WARFIELD,

Author of a "History of Imported Short-horns"; and a Staff Correspondent of "The Breeder's Gazette."

CHICAGO:

J. H. SANDERS PUBLISHING COMPANY.

1889

TO THE

CATTLE-BREEDERS OF AMERICA

THIS LITTLE BOOK IS DEDICATED

as a slight expression of appreciation of many kindly words and deeds.

PREFACE.

IN this little book I have endeavored to gather together such parts of my contributions to the periodical press for a number of years past as seemed to be of sufficient value for the practical breeder to justify a more permanent form. If an earnest effort to do something for my fellow-laborers in the great domain of cattle-breeding needs any justification, I may, perhaps, find it in the kind reception which my occasional writings have met with from the cattle-breeders of the country. I am grateful to them for many years of friendly appreciation, and I offer this digest of my work in the hope that it may prove of some value to them and to those who shall succeed them.

I wish to take this opportunity to acknowledge the assistance my sons have given me in preparing all my work for the press. Without their aid much—even most—of it could never have been done. Much of the work of prepar ing this book for the press has been done by my younger son, Ethelbert D. Warfield of Miami University. Great credit is also due to my elder son, Prof. Benjamin B. Warfield, D. D., now of Princeton, N. J., whose energy and vigor of thought and pen gave me such essential aid in the earlier years of my connection with the press; nor has the pursuit of the more weighty things of theology destroyed his capacity for taking an occasional part in the active discussion of cattle matters. The papers which have appeared over my signature have thus to quite a large degree been of family origin; and, as the time must come when I shall pass on both the work of writing and breeding to them, I am glad of an opportunity to make this acknowledgment of their filial aid.

WILLIAM WARFIELD.

GRASMERE, near Lexington, Ky.,
May, 1889.

TABLE OF CONTENTS.

PART I.—THE THEORY.

PART II.—THE THEORY APPLIED.

PART III.—THE PRACTICE.

PART I.—THE THEORY.

CATTLE-BREEDING A SCIENCE AND AN ART.

Reflective men have in all ages acknowledged the charm of agricultural pursuits, and, above all, of those which are especially concerned with the breeding of domesticated animals. They draw man's mind away from the daily vexations and cares of life to a contemplation of the course of Nature and those laws which God ordained in creation for the ordering and governing of the world. The cultivation of the soil and the raising of the annual crops which each season yield after their own kind teaches a dependence upon the higher power which controls the seasons and sends the sunshine and the rains of heaven in due proportion. To those who follow the avocations of this branch of agriculture there is little room for any other action than a close observation of natural laws and a wise and strict conformity to them. But in the breeding of live stock, of what kind soever it may be, while the observation of the course of Nature is no less important, there is, furthermore, place for the exercise of much higher faculties.

The stock-breeder has something more to do than merely to effect the coupling of one animal with another. To rightly fulfill the function of his calling he must so mate animal with animal as to produce the best possible results, generation by generation, in an ever-ascending proportion. To him are entrusted living organisms from which he is to produce, according to the natural laws of propagation, other similar organisms, and of such a character as shall conserve every good quality and as far as possible replace every bad quality with a good, or at least a better. These organisms are therefore plastic. The secret of their plasticity is not known to every one, and to those to whom it is known it is still a mystery, or at best a half-read riddle. In just the ratio of the insight that this man or that has into this secret of Nature will he become a successful breeder. This insight, in fine, is knowledge, and like all other knowledge it is power, and he that would possess it must seek for it as for hid treasure.

There may have been a time when men were ignorant of the value of this branch of knowledge; but if so it was beyond the first faint dawn of human history. The earliest written records of the race show that certain breeds of horses were already specially esteemed, and that the dog had been greatly specialized to meet the requirements of man in the pursuit of game and his other vocations. The pyramids of Egypt not only reveal at least three distinct types of the dog, of widely varying character, but they indicate that even in the hoary antiquity from which they speak cattle were esteemed for certain well-defined peculiarities, and it is scarcely an overbold corollary from this fact that the cattle were bred with a view to the special production of certain highly-esteemed marks. Thus we see how early man began to adapt the beasts about him to his uses, not merely by taming them but by breeding with a view to more and more perfect adaptation to his needs.

The early experiments were doubtless crude in the extreme, and yet it can scarcely be doubted that they were suggested by the appearance of that tendency to variation which, as will be seen in the course of this inquiry, has been such a potent factor in the whole history of improvement and specialization. These steps, therefore, feeble and tentative as they were, proceeded on firm ground and indicated a steady advance. It can hardly be doubted, however, that all such progress was in the main individual and in a great degree dictated by chance, or at most by an unorganized though rational seizure upon a windfall of fortune. The advance through many centuries was, therefore, except in a few instances, extremely slow and variable. Hence it is that we find although the classic writers of Greece and Rome reveal again and again the existence of improved breeds of various kinds of domestic animals, with few exceptions those animals existed at the beginning of the eighteenth century throughout Europe in a state which showed little or no advance over the breeds described by Pliny and Columella. Not that there was not then as now great variety in the breeds cultivated in different countries. Then a long-horned, ill-favored breed roamed the fair but infertile plains of Italy, while the low countries, that are the Holland and Belgium of to-day, possessed a breed that was the natural complement of their frugal and thrifty, if homely life. The hills of Wales then, as now, were occupied by a diminutive stock, while the rich uplands and luxuriant meadow lands of "Merrie England" raised, even then, cattle from which the feeder reared beeves whose carcasses were eaten with gusto in hall and tavern. But in every land it was the native stock, improved, if improved at all, only by the unconscious moulding of the national wants and needs. The Dutch loved cheese, the English beef, and the result was worked out in broad but in as yet indefinite lines in the cattle of the two countries.

But the eighteenth century witnessed a great awakening of interest in all agricultural affairs, and toward the last quarter of the century the neat cattle became a center of this interest. This was particularly so in England. And it is at this time that the general progress comes to have the first hero of its work. Prior to this time the improvers who added here a little and there a little to the quality of the stock they bred were never known, or if known were quickly forgotten. Robert Bakewell is the first name on the roll of the great improvers of English cattle. Besides other animals he gave great time and attention to the breeding and improving of the Long-horned breed. From his experiments sprang a long series of efforts for the improvement of English cattle. This movement was nearly synchronous with the general movement which brought all the appliances of science and the results of knowledge in every sphere into the work of increasing the productiveness of agricultural labors. Bakewell devoted himself to the study of breeding principles in a systematic and thorough-going way. He had little to build on. Natural science as we know it was almost undeveloped. He was a pioneer, and he did his work thoroughly and accumulated a mass of material in the results of many experiments which was the great foundation stone of later work.

It is not my purpose to even briefly sketch here the progressive steps by which the work begun by Bakewell grew into the fabric which we possess. Let it suffice to say that what he began others—both scientists and breeders—pushed on with well-directed labors, each adding his mite to the general sum of knowledge. My purpose is rather to point out that, while prior to the appearance of Bakewell there was little known in regard to cattle-breeding and little attention given to it, since his time it has risen so rapidly that it is perhaps not claiming too much to assert that there are both a science and an art of breeding.

Science is primarily knowledge, and secondarily it is knowledge systematized and arranged. For more than a hundred years acute observers have been gathering facts and studying the phenomena of animal reproduction. During this time an immense number of facts have been collected, collated and arranged with reference to the elucidation of the many problems affecting the transmission of life. Out of these investigations have grown many special studies of particular departments of the great general subject. Studies of the laws of heredity, of natural selection, and many other specific problems have won years of devoted labor from many active scholars. What the scientist has approached from the side of theory the practical breeder has assailed on the side of practical every-day utility. The studies of the one have borne their due fruit in the application of their results to the labor of the other, and the end is seen in the steady improvement of so many breeds of cattle.

It does not prove that there is no such thing as a science of breeding to show that the ordinary course of breeding cattle is controlled by no law or system of laws, that it is the result of no special knowledge, but is simply an unregulated and unordered progression. It is perhaps too true that the practice of a great many breeders is reducible to no system, and that Hap-hazard is the presiding tutelary God of their farms. But this does not prove anything against the existence of a science of breeding. It merely shows that if there is such a science it needs to be more widely taught.

It would perhaps be claiming too much to assert that this science is an exact science or a thoroughly systematized one. But there are few of which this can be said, and they are not those from which man derives the highest truth. In this life we must be content "to know in part." Perfect and absolute knowledge is not the prerogative of mortal beings. This science of breeding, then, is the systematized facts and the laws deduced from them whereby we are to be regulated in our practical work of breeding. It is, in short, the theory of breeding, and under that term I shall attempt so much of an account of it as seems to me useful to the practical breeder in his ordinary course of breeding.

Science is "knowledge systematized and arranged." A science is knowledge in some one department so systematized and arranged. So an art is defined by a high authority as the "application of knowledge or power to practical purposes." Thus we see that the art of breeding stands in the same relation to the practical side of the calling as the science does to the theory. If we have a science of breeding and breeders lay hold of the knowledge thus obtained and apply it to the daily problems which they meet, they may fairly claim for their work the dignity of an art. One of the useful arts it most truly is. Knowledge is power; knowledge or power, they are two different terms for the same idea, applied to practical purposes; applied to the breeding and developing of a breed of cattle—this, then, is the art of cattle-breeding.

I have said that the nature of animals considered in a wide view was plastic. This suggests a comparison with what are in common speech known as the plastic arts. Think of the potter moulding his vessels of clay; in the highest department of his art he has before his mind an ideal, and he works it out upon the clay in some beautiful shape and adorns it with some elegant design. If he be a true artist he will work long and faithfully, making many designs of exquisite loveliness, and yet never satisfying in a single instance the ideal in his brain. The world may applaud, he may himself feel conscious that he has done good work, true work, but never the highest and best that he had aimed to do. And yet how ductile the clay! How easily moulded to any shape by the cunning fingers under the direction of the eager brain! How receptive the blank surface of the finished vessel and how bright the colors ready prepared for its adornment! But he who breeds cattle has to do with living organisms; plastic, indeed; yielding strange and wonderful changes under the hands of some cunning artificer, now and again, whose masterwork is at once the admiration and despair of many contemporaries and successors. But even in his hands a thing so highly strung that the tense cord, if I may use a figure from another sphere, seems ready to snap even while it yields the purest strains. Many, even most breeders, seem never to learn how to breed the animal nature to their will. But there is no question that it can be moulded even as the potter's clay. Not so easily—only with infinite knowledge and skill. But the very nicety of the work, the very difficulty of the task, lifts the artist and his art at once to the highest plane. He who moulds the counterfeit of life may, indeed, be the artist of no mean art; but surely thrice greater he who with no less skill manipulates the complex nature of a living being, producing a superior form and one in conformity with the ideal in his mind. Such a view is far from exaggerated. The world is full of countless varieties of a single species of domesticated animals which are only modifications wrought out by man's ingenuity. The various breeds of cattle, horses, sheep, dogs, fowls, pigeons, and many other animals, not to speak of the infinite beauty and variety of the variations produced in the vegetable kingdom by the magic of man's skill, attest the marvelous extent to which man has moulded and is still moulding the domesticated animals.

The breeding of cattle is, then, if rightly followed, a true art. It may sink very low. The artist may be only a caricaturist. But if the knowledge and the power which are free to every man who chooses to make them his are properly applied the breeder will not be unworthy of the name.

The fine arts then are not all the arts. And even in the fine arts the final execution of some masterpiece is not all the art. The paints must be mixed, the canvas prepared, and many minute and often laborious and always prosaic things be done by the painter ere the first outline is traced upon the final canvas. The sculptor must seek his clay often at great trouble, must mould and model and toil at many a little and irksome task before he can think of the marble. There are no less many prosaic things in our breeding of cattle, and I shall write of many details that are important, if scarcely counted in the final sum. The cattle-breeder needs no one to tell him how many little trials he meets day by day, how many sore disappointments, how many things that make him think that he lives for the day and not for any high and noble end. What I have written here I have written largely with a view to call off the mind from this one view of the subject. It is a great help to rise above the little and narrow view and see the world from an entirely new and wider standpoint. How different the impression created upon the mind by a single landscape viewed from the level of the plain and again from some lofty mountain top! And so it is here. Not that I would have the plain, straightforward business aspect ignored. Wherever business relations enter the field they are honorable and of the highest importance. They are, however, not likely to be overlooked; they are too aggressive and thrust themselves too much on our attention. We are too little given to remembering that there are any other considerations except such as are closely reckoned in dollars and cents. I should prefer to regard the monetary return only as a fair and just standard whereby to gauge the judgment of the world on our work; and as we are prone to be very partial judges of our own work such a standard is not unlikely to measure in no inaccurate way our success in turning out art products. The world may, indeed, be deluded for a time into giving more for a poor beast than a fine one, just as it was into ranking Guido Reni with Raphael, and into giving $17,000 for the "peach-blow vase," but such aberations are rarely of long duration and will in good time right themselves.

And so in the following pages I propose to treat of the theory and practice of breeding in a plain and unambitious way, but I shall consider at the same time that I am treating of the science and the art of breeding; and while my aim is to prepare a manual for the farmer and breeder in his ordinary course of breeding and handling cattle I shall endeavor to present the subject in such a way as to show the scope and unity of it in its higher relations.

HEREDITY—THE BREEDER'S CORNER-STONE.

The great fundamental proposition in all questions of breeding is that "like produces like." On this basis, whether formulated in words or not, men have built from time immemorial. This fact forces itself on the human mind, must have forced itself on the mind of our first ancestors, as the normal condition of natural production. Every animal under ordinary conditions brings forth "after its own kind." This law runs through all Nature. "Do men gather grapes of thorns, or figs of thistles?" asked the Lord of his disciples, recognizing this law in the vegetable kingdom!

Had there never been any reason to believe that this great general law had some exceptions to its universal application it would probably have never been given any particular attention, and would have been passed over as too obvious to deserve more than a passing assertion unsupported by proofs and unillustrated by examples. It has become important, however, since the enunciation and development of the theory of variation, to bring out the normal action of this law, and to illustrate its scope and its general prevalence, in order to preserve due proportion in the explanation of the influences that are to be considered in breeding cattle.

Man must have recognized in the earliest times the law that "like produces like" as applied to man. The least observing mind would early have this truth forced upon it. How well fixed this was in the very earliest time of which we have any account is illustrated in all early records by the observed line of demarkation which personal appearance drew between different races. This was of course based on the knowledge that from Greek parents could spring only one having the Greek type of form and feature; and so also of Egyptian, Hebrew, Ethiopian, Accadian, etc.* Nor are the earliest literatures wanting in clear and distinct recognition not merely of this law as applied to the wide field of racial resemblances, but it is noted with respect to tribal, family, even personal resemblances. In these cases the law appears as a recognized fact—first as merely existing—it is not long till its power comes to be recognized as a means to an end. Men began to se-

* In the monuments of Egypt, for example, it is easy to trace the race types assigned to different dynasties even, the Hyksos or Shepherd kings being especially unlike native dynasties; and the Egyptian type is strongly distinguished from others, such as the Assyrian, Hittite, etc.; so also in the Assyrian and other monuments.

lect animals of like character and breed, then, with a view to preserve the type. Thus the Arabs, when scarcely more than half-wild savages, kept records of their horses' pedigrees and valued them scarcely less than such pedigrees are valued today. In the days of the Roman Empire so fully had this law come into general recognition that for the sport of the luxury-degraded people who had once by sturdy manhood achieved the mastery of the world all kinds of monstrous forms were cultivated and bred, showing that the world had already learned how broad the law was; that not only were normal characteristics reproduced but that abnormal features were also propagated; and that the rule was not merely general but that it extended to the reproduction in the offspring of many of the most trivial personal peculiarities.

A few particular examples may perhaps best make clear the great breadth and at the same time the minute influence upon detail which the power embodied in this law has. I shall begin with the more general and proceed to the more special cases.

Perhaps the most general type of cases are those of race peculiarities. The large-framed blonde type of the Teutonic peoples, the smaller dark-hued type of the Italian and other Southern races, the yellow of the Mongolian, the dusky, curly-haired type of the negro races; these all produce generation by generation the same type so long as kept pure; but when the blood of one intermingles with another an instant change to an intermediate type ensues.

Then we have well recorded instances of close resemblances in families for many generations. Thus the ill-fated house of Stuart was marked by a family resemblance of the most striking kind, one which the portraits of its members, even under the utmost efforts of court painters to "individualize" their "subjects," makes startlingly clear to us. In the families of Valois and Bourbon, too, ran a line of strong resemblances. Indeed, not only among ruling families, but wherever a long line of portraits have preserved to us a record of the personal appearance of a number of generations we find that in a large majority of cases there is a strong resemblance.

But this influence is not confined to mere externals; it goes to the deepest things of the mind and character. If the Stuarts were alike in form and feature how much more in that headstrong, incapable nature that could learn neither from precept nor experience! How plain bluff Hal shines out in good Queen Bess despite the powder and the patches with which so many generations have sought to hide the too palpable likeness.

And so Darwin quotes ("Animals and Plants Under Domestication," Vol. II, p. 25,) from an earlier writer the case of a man who was in the habit of sleeping on his back "with his right leg crossed over the left, and whose daughter, while an infant in the cradle, followed exactly the same habit, though an attempt was made to cure her." What may be considered an exactly analogous case has happened here in my immediate neighborhood. The celebrated race horse and great sire imported King Ban, owned by Maj. B. G. Thomas of Kentucky, had a singular trick of standing, even out in his paddock, with his fore legs crossed. Year by year it came to be noticed that the colts of his get in a singularly large number repeated this habit until it got to be a thing regularly looked for that quite a number of the foals of each year should repeat their sire's extraordinary way of standing. Their genial owner was very fond of calling attention to this circumstance as one of many striking illustrations of King Ban's power of impressing his get with his own characteristics.

As an extreme case of inheritance of a minor peculiarity I may cite a case which has come under my immediate observation of a gentleman whose hair grew in a peculiar manner on his brow and at the crown of his head, being what in common parlance is spoken of as very badly "cowlicked." This peculiarity was transmitted to a son, and through a daughter to two grandsons. This fact has been frequently alluded to in my hearing by two barbers who were in the habit of cutting their hair, and who complained that their heads were all alike and that it was impossible to get the hair of any one of them to lie down. A number of cases are reported of the transmission through a number of generations of a lock of hair colored differently — most generally white — from the rest of the hair; and I have known, in a family of close friends, of the transmission through several generations of a singular red mark down the center of the forehead, and which is casually spoken of as a matter of course as the "H—— blaze."

In respect to character and temper a number of proverbs, such as "like father like son," "a chip of the old block," and many others, attest the popular faith in the doctrine of heredity. It has come to be the common belief in this country that great men's sons are rarely worthy of their sires, but opportunity and education have so much to do with making men what we in this new world term great, that this argument cannot be pressed very far. That the sons of great men have sometimes preserved their birthright intact despite the snares of inherited greatness the annals of many countries prove.

One and twenty of the noble family of Scipio attained to consular rank, and it was a daughter of one of these who bore those brilliant orators and splendid friends of popular liberty the Gracchii. Among the lower animals the blood of such horses as Eclipse and Lexington, of Hambletonian and Denmark has shown not only power but immense persistency in shaping the three types of thoroughbreds, trotters, and saddle horses.

I might go on thus multiplying instances, of singular instructiveness in some cases, all pointing to the wide scope and the minuteness of influence of the transmission of individual or family peculiarities. But I must be content with the few I have cited, only pausing to call especial attention to the frequent abeyance in one generation of a quality peculiar to the opposite sex which at once appears in the produce of that animal of the contrary sex. This is surely a very beautiful illustration of heredity. No more apposite example can be given than that of Comet Halley Jr., a Short-horn bull of a good old family of excellent milkers, who carried on the milking qualities of his dam in a remarkable degree to his calves. Nor was he more than a very prominent example of a class. It is a frequent occurrence to see Jersey bulls advertised as "butter bulls," which shows the accepted view that bulls whose dams were butter cows will carry on the capability to the third generation.

We thus lay down the general thesis that "like begets like." It is now important that this proposition should be somewhat carefully analyzed. First, then, it follows without more proof that ordinary qualities are transmitted. Some of the examples show that even tricks and peculiarities of body and of mind are transmitted. It is, however, specially important to note that defects and diseases are reproduced with as great persistency and frequency as normal characteristics. This is a point of deep importance. The medical profession fully recognize it, and to the breeder it becomes a source of care and watchfulness.

Medical science recognizes the inheritability not merely of such diseases as consumption, scrofula, and others of kindred nature, of mental disorders such as lunacy and idiocy, of defects such as imperfect sight and hearing, but of many other obscure and faintly-developed peculiarities of body, temperament, and mental state. Deformities of every sort—abnormal growths of hair, of scaly dermal affections, and many like appearances—prove oftentimes highly hereditable.

Pulmonary complaints affect cattle no less than man, and are found to be quite as surely passed on from father to son. Other weaknesses of constitution, tendency to abortion, to early loss of fertility, and so forth, are the compensation to maintain an equilibrium, where, on the other hand, high flesh-making qualities and superior milking qualities are similarly transmitted.

A few observed instances of this hereditary nature of physical defects and diseases may not be out of place by way of arresting attention and exhibiting the very radical and far-reaching influence which they possess.

As illustrations of mere physical defects the well-known frequency with which persons who are left-handed pass on the defect to their children* may be considered as a limiting value, that is as on the border land between a mere habit and a physical defect. Darwin cites from "Anderson's Recreations in Agriculture," etc., Vol. I, p. 68, the case of a one-eared rabbit which produced a breed kept up for some time which possessed only a single ear; and also the case of a bitch which had a defect in one leg which was transmitted to her puppies. The widely-cultivated breeds of lop-eared rabbits and of Manx tailless cats offer other illustrations of

---

*Thus in the Biblical account of the tribe of Benjamin: "The Lord raised them up a deliverer, Ehud—a Benjamite, a man left-handed."—*Judges iii, 15.*

"And the children of Benjamin were numbered at that time. * * * Among all this people there were seven hundred chosen men left-handed; every one could sling stones at an hair breadth, and not miss."—*Idem xx, 15-16.*

this sort, and Darwin cites from a German authority the very strong case of a cow which, having lost a horn by disease, produced three calves which in lieu of a horn on the same side of the head as that from which their dam had lost her horn had only a "bony lump merely attached to the skin." Darwin suggests that this case approaches "the doubtful subject of inherited mutilations," but it is to be clearly noted that the mutilation arose from disease and not from mechanical means—a distinction of the highest importance.

Passing on to the class of cases where the cause is active and in the nature of disease we find such well-authenticated cases as the inheritance of ringbone, spavin, navicular disease, and similar affections in horses. These diseases are most frequently latent at birth, and only begin to develop as the horses reach maturity. Of this sort Miles, in his work on stock-breeding, cites the case of a mare that was affected with ringbone and incapacitated by it for work, but from which a number of colts were bred. Her colts at two and three years old showed no signs of the disease, but at five to six years they had all of them developed the disease.

Another well-known disease which is well recognized as hereditary among horses is roaring, and even more so ophthalmia. The Irish horse Cregan, of considerable celebrity, is reported (Dr. Finlay Dun in "Journal Royal Agricultural Society") to have transmitted the latter disease, which he had in a very violent form, to the fifth generation of his descendants, causing loss of sight at a very early age, one too early for them under ordinary circumstances to have contracted the disease.

But as already indicated pulmonary diseases and scrofulous complaints, such as consumption, diarrhea, dysentery, glandular swellings and suppuration, are peculiarly subjects of inheritance, and readily pass into what may be termed chronic hereditability; that is to say, become congenital. These diseases have been in man studied with great thoroughness as to their congenital character, and the great mass of statistics which have been gathered attest this character beyond a question. Nor is it less true of animals, and especially of cattle. I have known family after family of cattle which had congenital tuberculosis, and also not a few with scrofulous tendencies to glandular swelling and tumors. In some cases the organ affected will not be the same. As for instance, a cow will transmit a scrofulous tendency to tuberculosis to her calf, but while in her it affected the lungs in the calf it will affect the alimentary canal and take the form of consumption of the bowels or of chronic, malignant diarrhea. These are the diseases which the stock-breeder should be most strongly warned against, and the earliest possible moment should be seized for their extinction by slaughtering all the animals in whose veins flows the tainted blood.

And in these cases not less than in those where some healthy quality is transmitted it is not less usual for the disease or defect to skip a generation, or to pass from one branch to a collateral one in its appearance. Thus it frequently occurs in both consumption and lunacy that the alternate generations possess almost entire immunity from the disease; and again, that a father will transmit a disease to his daughters only in the first generation, but also to his son's children in the second. Many such irregular appearances are recorded. In some cases the disease seemingly having a co-ordination with a certain temperament or bodily peculiarity, as in one case where the disease, consumption, showed an affinity for a blonde type, while a brunette type about equal in number to the blonde possessed entire immunity. None of these manifestations of irregularity in transmission have ever been reduced to anything more than the few general classes which have been indicated. The subtle laws of this department of nature being as yet unknown.

Thus we see what consideration is to be attached to the inheritability of ancestral qualities. We have hitherto approached the consideration of this subject in a broad general view. It is now important to consider it from a more special standpoint with reference to the actual cases put to us in deciding upon a course of breeding. The first question that meets us is the relative value of the two animals at any time interbred. We have the two animals, and from their union according to the laws of procreation springs a third. This animal is a product of the parent natures, and our inquiry now is: in what proportion. The *prima facie* case is in favor of an equal influence of male and female. With no further data for our conclusion we are driven to accept the equal fusion as the only solution.

Many attempts have been made to show that one parent controls the external appearance and the other the disposition. Many more or less ingenious theories have been advanced taking almost every conceivable view; but I am unable to see that any advance of a tangible nature has yet been made. And until such is the case I think that we are justified in assuming that in the simple form of the proposition above given we are to assign equal weight to each parent as a factor in the product.

We have, therefore, with respect to the question of inheritance, to discover how the natures of the parents have mingled. It needs no argument to show how little we can tell of the result by even a full knowledge of sire and dam. It is as if two chemical substances hitherto never united were in our hands about to be combined. Who could prophesy that two parts of hydrogen gas and one of oxygen would form a drop of water? Let the bull stand for the two parts of hydrogen (H_2) and the cow be denoted by one part of oxygen (O), and interbred we would have a product (H_2O) composed of nothing but the two entities we once had whose character and nature we understood, and yet utterly inexplicable by anything known of the component parts. The skillful analyst can again resolve one drop of water into its original elements. A careful observer may in one case and another trace the lines where the two animals unite in their offspring, but not very often. The union of one animal nature with another is too intimate and too subtle to ever be clearly understood or sundered.

But in breeding cattle this much is certain: that each breeding animal must be weighed in the scale as one-half of every desired resultant. This is the basis of all our calculations. We shall see hereafter the special influences, such as animal prepotency, which often affect this calculation, and when once observed in any given animal, whether existing as a positive or negative quantity in the particular case in hand, it must be taken into account.

We see, then, that we must consider sire and dam equally as factors in the product we desire to obtain, and that each must be regarded as eminently likely to reproduce in the offspring not merely their form and nature in a general way, but that they will even stamp their image on the young animal in many smaller matters of detail. It would appear as if the animal were blocked out in the rough by a general union of the two natures and finished in all those elements which give individuality by a somewhat promiscuous borrowing of the details of feature and character of now one and now the other parent. It seems promiscuous and unordered because the laws which govern the methods of God's great laws that control these things are as yet unrevealed to us.

Let me borrow an illustration of how this intermingling would seem to be done from a new application of an old art—composite photography. The photographer takes upon his sensitive plate the portrait of a man, immediately upon this is superimposed that of another person, and so on indefinitely. In the end a picture is obtained in which those lines are very strong that occurred in every face, and each line is weaker in proportion to the number of faces which lacked it; and so on till the lines which occurred in only one face are faint and hazy, and float like a mellow mist about the picture made of the coincident lines. So every animal may be viewed as the sum of a large number of images of his ancestors. Every line in all their pictures is there; some so faint as to be of no significance, others merely suggesting the ancestor here and there. Others, where a number of tendencies unite on a single line, stand out and really give the animal its character. Where the lines of dam and sire lie one above the other the character of the animal may generally be traced. Where one is prepotent let us say that the first picture is printed very faintly, the last very heavily so as to almost obliterate the first faint lines. Again, let us say that one ancestor occurs a number of times in the pedigree of both sire and dam—that is, that his picture is taken in our composite photograph not once but repeatedly, so that its lines really are the chief factors in it. Will it be any surprise, then, to learn that the final composite is singularly like this ancestor? This is what is known in cattle-breeding as atavism, or reverting to an ancestor more distant than sire and dam.

But analogies must not be pressed too far. And we find that a single cross sometimes leaves so deep an impression in the blood that evidences will crop out again and again in remote descendants. But the special case of atavism demands more special treatment than can be given it in a remote allusion.

ATAVISM, OR REVERSION.

UNDER the name of "*atavism*" is now described what was once more commonly spoken of as "reversion," and in common speech as "throwing back"—*i. e.*, the special form of inheritance where the individual inherits some peculiar trait of a remote ancestor (Latin *Atavus*). We have had occasion already to notice some instances of this in the course of the general inquiry into the laws of inheritance. It is now necessary to briefly particularize.

Darwin says ("Animals and Plants Under Domestication," Vol. II, p. 41), in treating of this subject: "When the child resembles either grandparent more than its immediate parents our attention is not much arrested, though in truth the fact is highly remarkable; but when the child resembles some remote ancestor or some distant member in a collateral line, and we must attribute the latter case to the descent of the members from a common progenitor, we feel a just degree of astonishment." And while this is true and the mind that is not familiar with the singular and startling operation of the laws of "atavism" is often wonder-struck at the results, yet those who are familiar with the operation of that law—all who have had much experience in breeding animals of the same families for a number of generations especially—become so accustomed to the reversion to an old and long-unseen character as to regard such a reversion as a matter of course. The general recognition of atavism was probably first reached by agricultural students, though special cases were early recorded in human history. Indeed, there are few more striking instances of this law than that case recorded by Plutarch of the Greek woman who gave birth to a negro child, was tried for adultery, and was acquitted upon the proof that she was descended in the fourth generation from an Ethiopian. There is also an interesting passage in Thackeray's "Four Georges" (Vol. I, p. 4), in which he marks the reversion of George III to the character of an ancestor of the eighth generation—William of Luneburg—from whom he not merely inherited his blindness and insanity but also a number of the peculiar traits of mind and some of the special abberations of the old Duke. Writing of Duke William he says: "He was a very religious lord and was called 'William the Pious' by his small circle of subjects, over whom he ruled till fate deprived him both of sight and reason. Sometimes in his latter days the good Duke had glimpses of mental light, when he would bid his musicians play the psalm-tunes which he loved. One thinks of a descendant of his two hundred years afterward, blind, old, and lost of wits, singing 'Handel' in Windsor Tower."

Remarkable as this case is it is possible to more than parallel it with many instances of the highest authentication which have been recorded by breeders of various sorts of animals. One of the most noteworthy of these is that of a pointer bitch which at a particular time produced seven puppies at a litter, of which four were "marked with blue and white." This was so uncommon a color for the breed that it was supposed that some dog of another breed had had access to her and all the litter were marked for destruction, but the game-keeper was permitted to keep one as a curiosity: "Two years afterward a friend of the owner saw the young dog and declared that he was the image of his old pointer bitch Sappho, the only blue-and-white pointer of pure descent which he had ever seen. This led to close inquiry, and it was proved that he was the great-great-grandson of Sappho." (Darwin, "Animals and Plants," etc.)

But it is quite unnecessary to multiply instances. Under my own observation have come many cases. One class of cases which are specially frequent in Short-horn cattle is that of reversion to the colors of ancestors. This is so common as scarcely to deserve note when it occurs. I recall one instance, for example, where a red-roan bull was crossed on a well-mixed roan cow and the product was a perfectly white calf; and several similar cases where the calves were red, which, on the whole, is more remarkable since Short-horns exhibit a tendency toward light colors in many cases.

Mr. Darwin divides the observed cases as to animals under two principal heads: First, the reappearance of a lost character in pure breeds after a number of generations; and, second, the reappearance, where a cross has been made, of some peculiarity of the animal used to effect the cross which had not formerly occurred in the cross-bred descendants, or which had been early lost on a return to the use of a single strain upon the descendants of the cross.

Of the first class the not uncommon occurrence of small horns in well-bred Southdown bucks long after the breed had been bred to a hornless character is a widely-known example; while of the second an instance is recorded by Mr. Sidney, in his edition of "Youatt on the Pig," of a Berkshire boar being used on an Essex sow, the sows from which cross were bred to pure Essex boars, but twenty-eight years afterward a litter turned up containing two pigs of well-marked Berkshire characteristics. I have myself remarked in Kentucky how long after the total extinction of the Long-horn in this part of the world a calf would appear with the notable Long-horn mark of a white stripe down the backbone—a mark, I believe, peculiar to that breed.

From a cattle-breeder's standpoint this reversion to an archaic type is rarely a matter of much importance. It is of frequent occurrence in small things; thus, a black nose not infrequently crops out to the puzzle of the breeder till it is traced to a distant grandsire. Peculiarities of horn, of carriage, and many other similar features constantly admonish the close observer that "atavism" is a very real thing.

Not infrequently in a somewhat earlier day the breeders of polled cattle found this law of reversion a deterrent factor in their efforts to fix a hornless character on their breeds. It is now well settled that our polled cattle, certainly those of British origin, came from a horned type. The historical evidence, which for this purpose is almost conclusive, and the geological record agree upon this point with the greatest exactness. Long after the polled breeds of England and Scotland had become well recognized as distinct hornless breeds animals would appear of the most undoubted purity of blood with horns. The atavic character of such phenomena is obvious. Not only is this true of British breeds, but of other similar ones. Thus we are informed by a good authority that a polled breed in the Corrientes not infrequently produced animals with small, misshapen, and sometimes unattached horns.

In treating of this question of atavism I have purposely chosen to follow the line indicated by Mr. Darwin in the quotation made at the beginning of this chapter. He practically treats it as the reversion to some ancestor more remote than the grandparents. This is calculated to show the more extreme instances of the action of the law, and like all extreme cases these are especially valuable as illustrations. Other writers, however, make the term atavism to apply to all reversions to an ancestor more distant than the parents. Of these the French writer on heredity, M. Ribot, is an eminent example. In defining atavism ("Heredity," p. 166,) he says: "Whenever a child, instead of resembling his immediate parents, resembles one of his grandparents, or some still more remote ancestor, or even some distant member of a collateral branch of the family—a circumstance which must be attributed to the descent of all its members from a common ancestor—this is called a case of atavism." Under so broad a definition as this all those cases where a grandson inherits through his mother his grandfather's peculiarities of physical and mental character, and a granddaughter her grandmother's through her father, a most important division of the subject of heredity would be included. Nor are there wanting many and highly-instructive cases of an inheritance from a grandparent by a line of the same sex peculiarities of form and temper where the parent is a mere connecting link in whom the quality transmitted is latent, if in any true sense it can be said to exist at all. Of such a transmission we have instances in the descent of the great qualities of Chárles Martel (or the Hammer), through Pipin the Short, to Charles the Great (Charlemagne); of the celebrated Dutch marine artist William Vandervelde to his more distinguished grandson William Vandervelde the younger through a son who was an artist but of no repute; of the musical power of the elder Louis Beethoven to his grandson the famous Ludvig through an undistinguished son.

These cases are all upon a line of transition, and no doubt it is the same law that is acting through the whole series from parent to a remote ancestor. The important idea which at least for the purposes of the present inquiry it is desirable to present at this time is the sudden, unlooked for, and distinct reappearance after a long lapse of some character of a remote ancestor for the last few generations extinct. Hence it is best to adopt the definition laid down at the beginning of this chapter, and relegate the special inheritance of the traits of grandparents to an intermediate class.

I shall content myself for the present with quoting one further instance of atavic manifestation of a most remarkable character, and which is vouched for by high medical authority; if it were not that other similar cases are on record it would be quite incredible. It may be added that albinos are often thus produced at frequent intervals in some negro families. The story runs thus (Ribot, "Heredity," page 169,): "Two negro slaves living on the same Virginia plantation were married. The wife gave birth to a daughter who was perfectly white. On seeing the color of the child she was seized with alarm, and while protesting that she never had intercourse with a white man, she tried to hide the infant, and put out the light lest the father should see it. He soon came in, complained of the unusual darkness of the room, and asked to see the babe. The mother's fears were increased when she saw the father approach with a light, but when he saw the child he appeared pleased. A few days afterward he said to his wife: 'You were afraid of me because my child was white, but I love her all the more on that account. My own father was white, although my grandfather and grandmother were as black as you and I. Although we are come from a country where white men are never seen, still there has always been one white child in families related to ours.'" This child was afterward exhibited before the Royal Society in London by Admiral Ward, who bought her from her master. Cases of an exactly similar nature are on record, some of which occurred in Africa, beyond the possibility, it is claimed, of there being any deceit practiced upon the observers. Whether these cases trace to a distant and forgotten infusion of white blood, or to some phenomena akin to that which gives us albinos, or even to a true and concealed white cross immediately, they are very remarkable as cases of atavism or under the last supposition of an unusual effect of prepotency, the laws of which we are presently to examine.

PREPOTENCY.

We have seen that the ideal law of inheritance is an equal mingling in the offspring of the natures of the parents. This, however, is rarely to be met in practical breeding. For various reasons—greater vigor of race or individual character, for example, in one parent than the other—the ideal is seldom attained. The young animal nearly always shows a closer resemblance to one progenitor than the other. The facts are very many, and the classification of them is as yet incomplete and the deductions drawn from them tentative. Many theories have been advanced to explain the observed facts. But the incompleteness of the data upon which the speculations rest is well shown by the fact that the theories are conflicting and at times directly contradictory.

Out of this chaos of speculation and out of the immense number of observations made in the formulation and buttressing of the deductions of this and that class of thinkers a general skepticism as to such laws of special organic influence in all cases of a single character has grown up and the theories have largely given way to a general support of the doctrine long a favorite with stock-breeders of prepotency.

Prepotency is the superior influence of one parent over the other in determining the character of the offspring.

Prepotency is usually treated as (1) prepotency of breed, race, species, and (2) prepotency of the individual. The one is general and the other special, the same law plainly acting in the same way in both classes. The division, however, has a special and very real value to the stock-breeder.

No better illustrations of the operation of this law in both classes can be given than those afforded by cattle-breeding. Thus the Short-horn was early recognized as a breed having singular power of fixing its character on other breeds. Says Mr. Darwin: "The truth of the principle of prepotency comes out more clearly when certain races are crossed. The improved Short-horns, notwithstanding that the breed is comparatively modern, are generally acknowledged to possess great power in impressing their likeness on all other breeds." This faculty has been called by a recent writer "free power," from the readiness with which it is transmitted, and after many investigations and experiments he concludes that the Short-horn possesses this "free power" in a higher degree than any other breed of cattle. It is this quality which has given them such a great reputation for crossing with the common native cattle of many countries for the purpose of improving them either as beef or milk producers or as the general-purpose cow of the small farmer. So great is this influence on other breeds that the first cross often produces even from very inferior cattle a beast scarcely inferior to the best of the improved breeds. Indeed I have myself known prize animals in the show-yard that were by Short-horn bulls out of native or "scrub" cows. And when put to pure-bred bulls this excellence is maintained without perceptible alteration, and many of the most successful show animals in Great Britain and America have had very short pedigrees.

While this "breed prepotency" is thus in an eminent degree possessed by the Short-horns, among them certain animals exhibit the individual prepotent power in a high degree. Thus the bull Favorite (252), which Mr. Colling bred into his herd as deeply as possible, making as many as three successive crosses with him, was of great vigor and of great prepotency. Under my own observation have come some very notable cases. Thus in the fifty-seven years since the herd was founded at Grasmere in 1831 by my father there have been twenty-seven sires used upon it for a greater or less period. Out of these thirteen were marked successes and were for years used as stock bulls, and out of these six showed a high degree of prepotency. They were Oliver (2387), in use from 1833 to 1840; Goldfinder (2066), from 1836 to 1841; Cossack (3508), from 1841 to 1844; Young Comet Halley (1134), from 1844 to 1847; Renick 903, from 1847 to 1856; Muscatoon 7057, from 1866 to 1873; and Baron Butterfly 49871 from 1883 to 1887. These bulls were all animals of an unusual capacity for impressing their own excellence upon their get. Oliver, the first in the list, belonged to the old Powell stock and came to Kentucky at a time when Short-horn bulls were chiefly used for breeding cattle for the beef market. The steers of his get were famous for their size and their extraordinary capacity for taking on flesh, accompanied with the greatest fineness of bone. So great was their bulk and so great the fineness of bone that it was found almost impossible to drive them, as the custom of the day was, to the Eastern cities, which then as now were the great consumers of Kentucky beef. His breeding was no less excellent in his own harem, where the cows were Short-horns of the best strains. From him were bred a large number of prize-winners, all of which showed their descent very plainly. I have seen few, if any, bulls that were superior to him as a sire, but he was not remarkable for individual fineness.

He was, in truth, somewhat plain, but possessing some most desirable qualities, and it was the fact that he transmitted these often to an even higher degree than he himself possessed them which made him so valuable as a sire and so good an example of prepotent influence. Goldfinder, Oliver's younger contemporary and successor in the headship of the herd, was a very unusually fine bull and successful in the show-ring everywhere. He made a broad mark on the herd by the general excellence of his calves and won great repute by the phenomenal excellence and wonderful show-ring success of some of his get, chief of which was the cow Caroline. This cow was shown from the time she was a calf at many exhibitions and never once beaten. After Goldfinder came Cossack, a very fine bull of Booth breeding and the first to bring to many Kentucky breeders a true realization of the high excellence of Booth cattle. He was very prepotent and perhaps has honor enough in having sired Buena Vista 299, the sire of Mr. Renick's great cow Duchess, and thus grandsire of the great bull Airdrie 2478, himself a grand sire; and in being through Duchess the progenitor of the favorite line of Renick Rose of Sharons. Next Comet Halley Jr., or Young Comet Halley, as he is also called— a good bull and a good breeder, chiefly notable for his remarkable prepotency in getting milking stock. His calves were fine examples of the transmission of what are called "secondary sexual qualities"—that is, qualities by their very nature peculiar to one sex and a concomitant of that sex by an animal of the opposite sex. Comet Halley, the sire of Young Comet Halley, was deeply bred in milking strains, being by Frederick (1060), Mr. Whitaker's celebrated sire of milkers, and from the famous Nonsuch, or Golden Pippin, tribe of Mr. Colling, while on his dam's side he was sprung from the admirable milking strain of the Illustriouses. His breeding thus gives us an insight into the factors which go to build up the force of which prepotency is the manifestation. But to pass on, we find in Renick another animal excellent indeed, but by no means extraordinary himself, breeding with the utmost certainty and regularity cattle of really phenomenal character. I could readily name a long list of prize-winners sprung from his loins, such as Mary Magdalene, an unrivaled cow, massive and deep fleshed, whose ankle bones even when she weighed 2,225 lbs. could be spanned by an ordinary man's hand, and who bore her rather gaudy red-and-white coloring with the dignity of a perfect form; but it would in this place be a mere unspeaking catalogue. One instance I shall quote as a single example of his impressiveness as a sire.

My father had an old brindle milk cow with upturned wide horns, a coarse, mean brute, of the true "scrub" type. This cow was bred to Renick, and produced a red heifer calf of extraordinary quality. I was a young man in those days, and I told my father that I was going to take the old brindle cow's calf and beat all the pure-breds. Of this he was skeptical. But the calf grew out finely and proved invincible, being, so far as any could penetrate, of the most perfect Short-horn type.

After Renick came Muscatoon, with an interval of good but not specially notable sires. Muscatoon quickly gained for himself a National reputation. The herd had grown in numbers and repute so that this celebrated bull reaped much from the sowing of his predecessors. He was certainly phenomenal, not simply as a breeder, but in that his bull calves displayed a large degree of the same power. For that reason I have not included in this list 2d Duke of Grasmere 13961, his son by Grace, a Rose of Sharon cow, and used in the herd from 1874 to 1883, because his influence was little more than a continuance of Muscatoon's impression. It would be impossible to enumerate even a partial list of the prize-winners this bull got. His period fell at a time when there was great interest in cattle-breeding, when the exhibitions were thronged, and the whole country was acquainted with cattle matters. His reputation under these circumstances flourished, and such calves as Loudon Dukes 3d and 6th, Loudon Duchess 4th, Maggie Muscatoon, Jubilee Muscatoon, Duchess of Sutherland 6th, and many others spread it everywhere.

Under very different circumstances Baron Butterfly of the old Barmpton Rose family came into the herd's chief place. But though during the years that he was used cattle circles were deeply depressed he won a wide reputation. For evenness and absolute certainty that he would make his mark on his get he has rarely been equaled. Certain marks he almost never failed to transmit; so that it was scarcely difficult to pick out of a large number of cattle those sprung from him.

This somewhat extended account of personal experience seems to me valuable, as it illustrates out of a record of many years the way in which this prepotency of an animal manifests itself. Out of twenty-seven sires only five or six possessed it in a marked degree. Each one of those twenty-seven was chosen with the utmost care and prevision, with a view to securing not only high merit but fine breeding capacity. Thirteen were successful breeding bulls, but all except those named did not make a strong and nearly invariable mark on their get. When bred to cows of vigorous constitution the offspring was as likely to show a clearly mingled likeness or a decided likeness to the dam as to the sire. The few had so great power of procreation in the line of the general rule that "like begets like" that it was wonderful that a calf did not resemble rather than that it did resemble them.

It is easy to trace the lines of prepotency in many well-known and thoroughly authenticated cases. One of the most notable is to be found in the singular resemblance preserved for many generations in the house of Hapsburg, for so long the reigning house in Austria. This resemblance, preserved in spite of foreign and often totally unrelated marriages, has excited the comment of the most unobservant. A number of similar cases have been remarked in the noble families of Rome, and it is not possible for any one with any faculty for observing likenesses to view the long lines of portrait busts which throng the galleries of Rome without receiving a lively impression of the strong resemblances, often persisting for many generations, in the families whose successive generations are there preserved to us in their portraits.

Passing from man we find that in the horse the influence of prepotency is not only recognized and highly valued, but the personality of it has been carefully distinguished. Thus the horses Touchstone and Launcelot, though full brothers, were as different as possible in the stud. The get of Touchstone revealed their paternity in a striking way, while Launcelot was very wanting in impressiveness: "The Touchstones have been mostly brown or dark bay, and as a lot have shown a high form as race horses; while the Launcelots have been of all colors and below mediocrity on the turf."* In America the name of Lexington, himself long since laid away beneath his native blue-grass sod, is still a power in the Thoroughbred studs, and some more recent sires, such as Longfellow, King Ban, and others, have had wide celebrity for prepotency. Among trotting horses, such animals as Rysdyk's Hambletonian, Mambrino Patchen, Pilot Jr., George Wilkes, and others, have displayed this power in a highly remarkable degree. It is a task only for a tyro to trace the blood of the Hambletonians and the Patchens when once pointed out, even among a large number of promiscuously-bred horses. The indications extend to resemblances in color, form, gait, temper, vigor, endurance, and every conceivable quality. The influence exerted by these sires was truly remarkable in their own get, and the way in which their get have maintained and perpetuated them greatly heightens the wonder with which we regard them.

* "Stonehenge" on "The Horse," quoted in Miles' "Cattle-Breeding."

Another instance of this power is to be found in the breed of saddle horses, which trace their high excellence to the Thoroughbred horse Denmark. He was celebrated for his saddle qualities, and begat a large number of animals of the same excellence. They in turn being largely used in the stud produced a profound, almost a transforming, effect on the saddle horse of Kentucky. "Stonehenge" parallels the case of Touchstone and Launcelot by a very striking instance of individual difference in breeding in greyhounds. The dogs Ranter, Gipsey Prince, and Gipsey Royal, highly-bred and widely-used stock dogs, though full brothers produced stock "as different as possible."

An interesting case is given where a ram of "a goat-like breed of sheep" from South Africa was bred to ewes of twelve different breeds, and in every instance the offspring were "hardly to be distinguished from" the sire. This striking case is probably to be ascribed to the class of race prepotency, and was doubtless the result of the vigorous, wild nature of the ram. A valuable experiment recorded by that learned French investigator, to whom all students of natural science owe so much, Girou de Buzareingues, throws additional light on the same class of cases. Two breeds of French sheep were crossed with the Merino by putting Merino rams to generation after generation of the French ewes and the resulting cross-bred ewes. The two breeds gradually yielded up their character, but one much more readily and rapidly than the other, showing a marked difference in the native vigor of the two breeds.

But it is surely not necessary to multiply examples. What has already been said is certainly ample to found those applications to practice on, which will presently be made, and to convince every one that to secure the best results in breeding cattle for market, bulls must be used from breeds of marked prepotency; and that in breeding cattle of pure breeds there is a wide difference in the value of individuals; and that for the highest results bulls of the greatest prepotency are to be sought. That is all that could be hoped for. So great a master as Darwin recognizes the difficulties in anything more than an experimental recognition of prepotency, and says: "On the whole the subject of prepotency is extremely intricate, from its varying so much in strength, even in regard to the same character in different animals, from its running either differently in both sexes, or, as frequently is the case with animals, * * * much stronger in the one sex than the other, from the existence of secondary sexual characters—from the transmission of certain characters being limited by sex —from certain characters not blending together—and perhaps occasionally from the effects of a previous fertilization on the mother. It is, therefore, not surprising that everyone hitherto has been baffled in drawing up general rules on the subject of prepotency."

VARIATION.

In the foregoing chapters I have endeavored to give a brief statement of the law of heredity, and to illustrate the more important special cases which occur under it. Even in the discussion of the law and of its operation it was evident that somewhere in Nature there was a contrary force at work. What that is will now be explained.

If the law of heredity always operated with perfect precision and equal force the results of breeding would be simple, and could always be expressed by a mathematical formula. But we have already seen that the normal condition even is not an equal admixture of the parents' natures; that this is purely theoretical and ideal. The force of heredity under what may be termed, perhaps not inaccurately, abnormal circumstances, we have had illustrated in the subordinate laws of atavism and prepotency. The exceptions to the rule of heredity, the power of darkness warring against the law of light, the world-born tendency of chaos in open opposition to heaven-born law and order, now require our attention.

The fact that Nature sometimes departs from

a right line early forced itself on the notice of man. Monstrous births of man and beast find a place in many of the early records of our race. The causes of these departures from the law of reproduction, from the rule that "like produces like," were, however, long in being inquired into in a scientific spirit. At first monstrous births were looked upon as evidence of the anger of the gods, and were regarded as portents of impending evil. In time, however, reason triumphed over superstition, and close investigation showed that these notable and awe-inspiring monstrous offspring were only the extreme and most radical cases of a large class which were occurring more or less frequently at all times in the animal and vegetable kingdoms. In short it came to be seen that in Nature there is a tendency to change from the ancestral type under certain conditions. This is more than a tendency to strong individualization which some have been inclined to reckon it. It differs in kind rather than degree, though often very similar to such a strong individualization. It may be defined as a tendency to variation from the parental type. Hence, it is usually spoken of as "variation."

The causes of variation may be in a very loose way classed as general, as affecting the whole number of ancestry and produced by gradual and long-continued influences; and special as affecting a single individual, and that often suddenly and at a known time. Thus the latter case is well illustrated by such paroxysmal occurrences as monstrous births of deformed, diseased, deficient and dwarf animals resulting from a sudden shock to the mother when pregnant. Perhaps to the same class are to be referred those cases where the mother's imagination has been deeply impressed at the time of impregnation, and sometimes even marking the offspring with some deformity corresponding with the subject of this mental impression. It has been known for many centuries that deformities, imbecility and other defects in the offspring were caused by the mother receiving during pregnancy a sudden fright or being stricken with grief, and that the resulting defect was very likely to be transmitted to posterity. One of the most frequently cited instances of the persistency of a suddenly acquired peculiarity of this sort is that of Lambert, "the porcupine man," whose skin was covered with "warty projections which were periodically moulted." His six children and two grandsons were similarly affected, and the peculiarity was observed for at least four generations, occurring only in the males among his descendants. The instance recorded in the book of Genesis of Jacob's device to secure a large number of kids which should be "ring-straked, speckled and grisled," is perhaps the earliest clear recognition of the influence of imagination at the time of conception on the dam. One of the most striking instances—one however, which may be either classed as the effect of imagination at the time of conception or during pregnancy, or as the combined result of both—is that set out in the following statement made by Mr. John B. Poyntz of Maysville, Ky. "In the month of July, 1863, the cattle," a lot of Alderney heifers and a bull—none of which "were marked or branded, nor were their ancestors" after 1850—"were placed in a woodland pasture well provided with water and blue-grass, and in the pasture were placed a number of Government horses for a period of several weeks. Each and every horse was branded on the lower part of the left shoulder with the letters U. S. In the spring and summer of 1864 the heifers had calves. One of the number produced a fawn-colored or reddish calf, and on the lower part of the shoulder were the letters U. S., formed of white hairs, plainly to be seen by casual observers, and shown by me to friends and visitors. In due time my U. S. heifer had a calf, which was marked with U. S. on the same place as her dam. The letter S. was not so perfectly formed as on the dam, but was too plain to be taken for anything other than the letter S. In the growth of these cattle or cows the letter moved higher up on the shoulder and appeared to elongate, and in five or six years the character or form of the letter was lost and appeared only as numerous small white specks or spots." This statement, together with those of a number of other persons, was published in the Maysville *Bulletin* a number of years ago. From my personal knowledge of Mr. Poyntz there is no question in my mind of the truth of his statement.

I shall not attempt to trace the action of the mental and emotional nature on the uterine system, and to show how or why the impression is created. Some writers boldly, on *à priori* grounds, reject the idea that such cases are in any wise connected with the causes assigned and refer them to the too common fallacy, *post hoc ergo propter hoc.* The arguments most often used against the causal connection of frights and mental impressions with peculiarities in the fœtus are based on the fact that such occurrences take place in a very small number of cases proportionate to the number of pregnant animals whose mental and emotional natures have been acted on during pregnancy. Negative arguments of this sort are utterly valueless. The cases which occur are confessedly extraordinary. The sudden checking of the regular flow of the blood to the fœtus or the arresting of the regular action of the secretory organs of the maternal system may not improbably show its effect. The effect of anger on the milk of a nursing woman, making it unhealthy and even poisonous to the child, is well known, but the cause is utterly undiscovered. So here. In some cases, as that of the mental shock of the murder of the favorite Rizzio under the eyes of the pregnant Mary Queen of Scots upon the future James I of England, then *in utero*, the result is co-ordinated with the cause; James' fear and shrinking from weapons and conflicts being the natural offspring of such a shock. Similar cases are recorded where women have been frightened by a one-armed or one-legged man, and produced children having similar defects. But the far larger number of cases are those in which the mark upon the child has no connection in appearance with any outward semblance of the cause or instrument of the shock or mental impression. The mark runs from a mere mark, such as a strawberry blotch—a frequent concomitant of shocks of grief or sorrow under my own observation—up to horrible deformities. Some years since a very brutal rape was committed in Lexington, Ky., and thence sprang a child of the most horrible deformity, the horror and dread of every one who passed through that part of the city where the child lived.

But it is in the class of cases first above

named that the chief importance of the laws of variation centers. The causes of general variation are many and often obscure. They are often the long accumulated force of years suddenly unloosed; they are sometimes the long continued attrition through generations of unfortunately situated individuals. Changed conditions, of climate, soil, food, or environment of any sort is then one of the great causes, hence the great cause of change which we are able to observe in domestication, involving as it does in many cases the most radical changes of environment. It is quite impossible to do more than indicate in outline some of the more notable facts connected with the operation of these causes. They are chiefly important to the cattle-breeder on account of two phases. First, the development of a new and valuable quality by taking advantage of the operation of this law; and second, the encouragement of the tendency to the loss (atrophy) of some existing feature which is deemed undesirable where the law is operating to destroy it; or the checking of this action by the proper change of conditions of life where the feature that is being atrophied is desirable. As examples of these cases we may take the Jersey, Holstein, and Hereford cattle. In the Jersey by choosing an artificial method of feeding, the breeders of these cattle developed to an abnormal condition the production of milk rich in butter fats. The Holstein by a similar treatment directed to the production of milk containing a large amount of cheese-making products (caseine) were carried to another special end. The Hereford was driven to a high stage of beef production under a specialized treatment. In each case the intense stretching of the line in one direction produced a counter effect by a partial loss of neglected qualities; of beef production in the Jersey, of that and also of fats in the abundant and caseine-rich milk of the Holstein; of milk production in the Hereford. A different course was early adopted by the breeders of the Short-horn (Durham) and they have always sought to develop this breed by careful selection to a high excellence as beef and dairy cattle, neglecting neither meat, milk, butter nor cheese-making qualities, and carefully guarding against the atrophy of any desirable quality.

"We have good grounds for believing," says Mr. Darwin, "that the influence of changed conditions accumulates, so that no effect is produced on a species until it has been exposed during several generations to continuous cultivation or domestication. Universal experience shows us that when new flowers are first introduced into our gardens they do not vary; but ultimately all, with the rarest exceptions, vary to a greater or less extent." He quotes with approval M. de Jonghe, who says that "There is another principle, namely, that the more a type has entered into a state of variation the greater is its tendency to continue doing so; and the more it has varied from the original type the more it is disposed to vary still further." What is here said of plants is as far as observed true also of animals, and the poet not only has not exaggerated, but rather understated the case, who says:

> "The grapes which dye [our] wine are richer far,
> Through culture than the wild wealth of the rock;
> The suave plum than the savage-tasted drupe;
> The pastured honey bee drops choicer sweet;
> The flowers turn double and the leaves turn flowers;
> * * * * * * * *
> The wild flower was the larger—[we] have dashed
> Rose blood upon its petals, pricked its cup's
> Honey with wine, and driven its seed to fruit,
> And show a better flower if not so large."

All variation, of course, is not toward improvement. It is by selection of those variants which exhibit more desirable qualities than the parent stock and inter-crossing them that these improvements are effected. Variation in a wild state is often retrograde. Seed that has fallen upon an unkindly soil is sure in a few generations to begin to vary for the worse. It is only by the closest watchfulness that man can keep up many of the highly-esteemed, improved varieties of animals and plants. In these cases man has developed, built up, changed, and by his interference he has introduced a new element of artificial life and dependence upon man into their natures. If this support were withdrawn the retrograde movement would speedily begin. Watch the summer fields and see how much more lusty the weeds grow than the corn, the cockle than the wheat. And the ignorant, seeing how quickly deterioration takes place in wheat that is run wild, stamped their recognition of this tendency by attributing to the wild rye, or "cheat," the character of degenerate wheat. In the economy of Nature the ordering of these relations of life is the same as under domestication, if not so obvious. By "natural selection" the strongest are made stronger; the weaker go to the wall. The survival of the fittest was a well chosen and apt term to express this idea. On some soils one plant will thrive and displace others which would displace it in a different soil. In one climate one variety of animals finds a congenial home while others pine and die.

But Nature is a cherishing mother. She knows the pangs of parturition too well to destroy a race of children which only need to be modified to meet new conditions of life. Hence, we see many animals and plants which after enduring changed condition of life for some generations suddenly begin to vary; that is, to try to adapt themselves to their new circumstances. Sometimes where nutritious food is less easily obtained the animal deteriorates, but is at the same time better adapted to its surroundings; again, where nutritious foods become more abundant a corresponding change for the better occurs. The Shetland ponies well illustrate this. They are perfectly adapted to their bleak and barren habitat, and this adaptation is certainly due to a deterioration from a larger and more active and more elegantly formed beast. The coarse bone, specially notable in the disproportionately large and ill-formed head, shows this, and they have developed a thick suit of wool in addition to the natural coat to protect them against the extreme cold, which comes on in the autumn and is early shed as spring deepens into summer. Imported into warmer climes these ponies in a few generations show a tendency to increase in size and lose the auxiliary coat of woolly hair. Wherever an animal or a genus finds it possible to adapt itself to its changed conditions it does so and survives, but many become extinct. We have in the geological record some remarkable examples of efforts on the part of animals to adapt themselves to such changes. Thus a mollusk family which was once very abundant, but which is now very rare, has left a wonderful record of its extraordinary efforts to maintain itself. The early forms of this mollusk inhabited a slender tube often of very great length, as for example the orthoceratite, which is a common Silurian fossil. In later times the more highly developed species were closely coiled, the highest of all being the still existing but rare "pearly nautilus," commonly known as the "paper sailor." For a great period the conditions seemed highly favorable to this family, and many beautiful species are preserved in our rocks. But a time came when the world had ceased to smile on them. The beautiful spirals then began to uncoil; some straightened out almost to the straight tube of the first ancestral type, and from this to the close coil almost every imaginable modification has been found. It was a brave fight plainly enough, but a vain struggle against an unkind fate.

It logically follows that such variations as are produced by an effort at adaptation to new surroundings would be likely to reproduce themselves upon the descendants of the animal in which it exists. In the variations of the class first treated of there is no such marked logical basis for persistence, since when bred back to animals of the ordinary form of the species the whole force of inheritance would militate to eradicate it. But even in these cases the malformation or other variation shows oftentimes a prepotency over the normal. In the cases resulting from the effort of Nature to adapt the beast to its surroundings the prepotency is more marked, so much so that it is one of the accepted principles that "a variation is prepotent over a normal characteristic." The variations being here the result of an accumulated tendency of a long period, often of many generations, not unnaturally show great strength and persistency.

As we have seen, there is no rule by which we can measure the amount of prepotency in any given animal or of any given tendency. Some variations occurring singly are naturally difficult to fix. Others occur contemporaneously in more than one animal, and these interbred give a starting point. In the breeding of pigeons the great field outside of the vegetable kingdom for the study of variation, selection and other natural laws, many new and peculiar varieties have been obtained by somewhat random crosses from which variations of many kinds have been secured and great numbers of extraordinary varieties obtained, all of which breed perfectly true.

The frequent boast of the breeders of polled breeds of cattle that when crossed with the horned breeds a great majority of the young cattle are hornless is a good illustration of this prepotency of the variation over the normal type, which is the more notable when taken in connection with the fact already cited that, at least down to very recent times, few herds, of however pure descent, failed to show an occasional sport reverting to the horned type from which they sprang.

It is important to observe that where variations occur they rarely affect a single organ, but to a greater or less extent the whole body, and it is particularly noteworthy that certain organs are in very close and intimate relations with each other, and that a change or modification of one is either accompanied by or quickly followed by a similar one in the other. This is no cause for wonder to any one who has studied the beautiful adaptation in all animal life of means to end, of organ to function. The all-wise Creator, in His infinite foresight,* has thus bound up every organism in the threads of a system which is not to be raveled out by man, but which may be viewed in its perfect harmony in such studies as this. Observe the correlation of stomach and teeth in all animals; compare the rodents and the ruminants, for instance, in this respect. These major organs of close and obvious functional relations are easily seen as united by a close bond. Many other and unexpected examples of correlation have been observed. "Thus pigeon fanciers have

* For a fine discussion of "Design," as applied to this subject, see the Duke of Argyle's "Reign of Law."

gone on selecting pouters for length of body, and we have seen that their vertebræ are generally increased in number, and their ribs in breadth. Tumblers have been selected for their small bodies, and their ribs and primary wing-feathers are generally lessened in number. Fantails have been selected for their large, widely-expanded tails, with numerous tail feathers, and the caudal vertebræ are increased in size and number." Among cattle we find that the hair and horns are correlated; so also the color of the face and the extremities; and some have thought that the circulatory system has something more than a mere physiological effect on the hide, being correlated with it; the connection between color of the hide and of the hair is well settled. An effort was at one time made to show that the connection between the milk glands and the nutritive organs were thus correlated. That is, that if the milk glands were largely developed it would so affect the organs of nutrition as to prevent the rapid accumulation of flesh. Perhaps a more accurate statement of this view would be that the milk glands and the organs of flesh-production were in a three-fold bond with the nutritive organs, which so acted as to prevent a development of cattle in a high degree as both milkers and beef-makers. The correlation of course being something more than the ordinary physiological connection. Now it is a matter of common observation that a special shape of the whole beast is typical of the two kinds of cattle. The beef type is the blocky, square-framed animal; the milk type, on the other hand, is wedge-shaped, with the base to the rear, and tends to angularity. In these types are to be seen well-marked types of correlation. But it does not follow, and here was the fallacy of the old theory, that because an animal bred for milk alone would gradually assume one type, and one bred for milk alone another, that the two qualities could not be compositly produced in a single animal; least of all, that the organs of nutrition were appositely correlated with the organs of beef and milk production, which was the thesis sought to be maintained. On the contrary, it is obvious that both milk and beef production are co-ordinate functions of the animal body. and that while one may be abnormally developed at the expense of the other, the natural state is one of balance. The mother that is herself beefy if unprovided with enough milk to keep a thrifty calf, indeed, almost negatives thereby the chances of the calf's growing into a deep-fleshed animal by imposing upon it a calfhood of insufficient nutriment. Of course in an artificial life the owner provides against this by nurse cows and other means, and so maintains a race of non-milkers. I am inclined to believe that Jersey calves allowed all their mother's milk till eight months old would produce in a few generations cattle inclined to vary to a higher type of beef cattle; excessive nutriment being the great cause of variation, as floriculturists and horticulturists have wonderfully shown.

But I shall not multiply instances of correlated variation, nor shall I go more deeply into this great, complex, and inadequately understood subject. We have seen that under changed conditions of life all animals tend to vary; that such variations as are thus produced may be made permanent by selection; that such a variation is prepotent over a normal characteristic, and is generally complex rather than single, affecting more than one organ, and that certain organs are so intimately related that any modification of one is accompanied or followed by a modification of the other.

PART II. THE THEORY APPLIED.

APPLICATION OF THEORY TO PRACTICE.

I HAVE always placed the highest possible value on a thorough understanding of the great natural laws of reproduction. I have, therefore, dwelt upon them at great length, and yet have only outlined them. I could wish that all breeders of cattle could have the inclination, time, and opportunity to master the investigations of Darwin, Lucas, Ribot, and a host of other careful students and laborious collectors of facts in this field. But we must be content for the present with what we have in hand and proceed to examine the applications of these laws to the practical principles of breeding. The true aim of every enterprising breeder is to hold fast to the good and stretch forward toward the better—progressive conservatism in fine. He must maintain the good which came into his keeping; if possible he will improve upon it.

The pole star of the breeder's career is, therefore, the law that "like produces like." By it he steers under all ordinary circumstances. Ordinarily speaking, then, the breeder expects to have his stock breed like themselves; breed "true," as the colloquial expression is. This is the sum of the hopes and expectations of a large majority of breeders; and we shall see in the course of this study that the principal value, as breeding cattle, of thoroughbred* varieties is that by having been long bred to a definite standard they have attained a fixed type from which they rarely depart, and may in consequence be trusted to "breed true," and also that the fundamental idea of "pedigree" is a guarantee of fixedness of character with a high standard.

The breeder next advances to the law of prepotency, and applies it principally by seeking an animal possessed of it for the head of the herd, thus endeavoring to fix his good qualities on all of the produce of the herd. In choosing a breeding bull no wise breeder can afford to neglect a careful study of his capacity as a breeder. A fine animal of high prepotent influence is one of those rare discoveries which go to make men successful above their fellows; and the advent of such a lord into the harem is oftentimes an epoch-making event.

The average breeder has little to do with atavism in practice except in a negative way, for while he may meet frequent instances in which it will show itself, it is not regular in its action and cannot be embraced in any calculations for the future.

---

*I use this word in the sense now so commonly given to it of purely bred.

The laws of variation, on the other hand, are always to be kept in mind. Variations are, perhaps, rare; when they occur they doubtless are not of a radical type in our old and well-established varieties. But variations do occur, and occur sufficiently often, and are sufficiently definite to merit careful attention and to encourage the thoughtful breeder to make the most of them. In the more recently improved breeds—in the grade and "scrub" and crossed cattle—variation takes place more often. But however these laws may be regarded as abstract and theoretical, the practical experience of almost any observant breeder will quickly convince the most skeptical that it is of the utmost importance that these laws should be understood, not perhaps in the sense that every breeder should be able to define and explain them, but rather that however formally unrecognized, yet that they should be practically acted on. The difference between the man who weighs well the rules and laws of Nature in the light of his experience, with a full knowledge of all that has ever been written on the subject, and he who, recognizing simply that a bull breeds like himself in proportion as he is vigorous, lusty, and well bred, selects in consequence a bull of these qualities, and of the highest degree of excellence obtainable, to use on his herd of fine cows, is much the same as the difference between six and a half a dozen. The existence and operation of the same laws are recognized in both cases. The fact that one man formulates, after a thorough analysis, the end and the means to reach it, while the other merely acts on the rules of his experience, which were no less real though never distinctly recognized except in a very general way, does not have the least significance. We shall see presently that the very first practical question presented to the breeder involves a knowledge of these laws of procreation. It is possible, of course, to breed cattle in a haphazard, unregulated way, taking little or no thought for the morrow and letting the present take care of itself. With such methods we have nothing to do. My effort is to address to the practical, wide-awake American farmer a treatise which will give him the light of years of study and experience, and to do what I can to encourage intelligent and well-considered habits of breeding.

INBREEDING.

One of the first problems which presents itself to the cattle-breeder is, What definite plan shall be followed in order to secure the best results? Nature's method seems to be a wide and general system of selection, in which the strong and vigorous are the winners and the weaker are crushed out. Among wild cattle the more lusty bulls have their choice of the cows in a way that under natural selection insures the best results to the race. No data under these circumstances can possibly exist as to how closely or how remotely such animals are interrelated, except it were in some few isolated and unimportant cases where a few animals may have chanced to be secluded from their kind. Under the normal wild state the tendency, estimated by the laws of "average," would be to maintain a nearly perfect balance year in and year out, generation after generation. If the conditions of life should suddenly change the result on such wild cattle would be to deteriorate or to improve the average according as the change was for their advantage or disadvantage. It is quite apparent that no question of breeding intrudes itself here. Nature's selection, while always in favor of the maintenance of the animals in the best manner, yet is impartial, and under ordinary circumstances would maintain an average. But under the well-known theory of averages, while the far greater number of cases fall at or near the average line, at the same time some will fall quite far away, and as many will exceed as fall short, and the extreme variation up and down will be equal. Say, for instance, that the average height of men in America is five feet six inches, then it follows that there are as many men over as under that height, and that the same is true with relation to two lines of equal distance from the line of average above to below—that is, there will be as many men under five feet as over six. It is not necessary to discuss at length the laws of "averages" and of "deviation from an average," these two propositions are now so well settled. We have, then, this first proposition, that all animals, under ordinary circumstances, will in a state of nature maintain the same average, and also that there will be a deviation of considerable extent above and below the average and of equal degree and extent both ways.

Let man interpose and domesticate a number of animals of one kind and Nature's laws are at once set aside. Naturally, those deviating furthest below the average are first disposed of, thus at once raising the average; then the males of highest deviation upward are selected to breed from, and under the idea that "like produces like" we are justified in expecting a further elevation of the average; and if a still further selection is made on the same basis, rejecting all bad and choosing only the best males to breed from, the improvement should be steady and should continue generation after generation. But throughout this process the tendency is by rejecting many inferior animals to reduce greatly the number of animals taken into our calculations. If we started after our first rejection with only a few very choice animals we would soon be brought face to face with the question as to whether we shall or shall not practice breeding of closely-related animals to each other. This is the exact problem which most improvers have had to solve as a living, assertive question which could not be evaded.

A few cows being chosen, and the best obtainable bull used on them, in many cases phenomenal results were obtained. Now and again a bull would turn up so superior as a breeder that it would seem as if it were a step backward to breed his get to any other bull except their sire or one of their brothers. Improvers of a number of breeds found that this method fixed and perpetuated the superior qualities which had been obtained, and many of them set a plain and intentional example of close, even highly incestuous breeding. The problem which they left to posterity is, Was this course an extraordinary one demanded by exceptional circumstances, or was it a general course commended and approved by the wise men of olden time for ordinary conditions, and consequently a valid precedent?

Thus we find Robert Bakewell, the celebrated improver of Leicestershire sheep and Longhorn cattle, breeding very closely. Bakewell is the typical eighteenth century improver. Before his time many experiments were made; but the great idea which prevailed in the earlier time was that crossing of different breeds was the road to improvement. Bakewell struck out along the then novel line of careful selection from a single variety or breed. He began his work by selecting the most completely distinct lines of blood to be found among Longhorns, and the best obtainable animals of those strains. Mr. Webster of Canley, in Leicestershire, probably had the best herd of Longhorns in England, and from this herd Bakewell obtained two heifers, and then he brought a "promising" young bull out of Westmoreland. From this small beginning he built up his famous herd. The produce of these three animals were crossed and intercrossed; but, to quote Youatt, "as his stock increased he was enabled to avoid the injurious and enervating consequence of breeding too closely 'in and in.' The breed was the same, but he could interpose a remove or two between the members of the same family. He could preserve all the excellencies of the breed without the danger of deterioration."

We see that he first selected the best obtainable animals of absolutely unrelated stocks; they were said to belong to two "branches" of the Longhorn breed; from these he bred very closely at first, and then as the number of animals increased he made the relationship of the animals as distant as possible within the limits set. Other breeders used his bulls, but he clung to his original families. This course resulted in the most absolute concentration of blood, as all lines ran to the three original animals. Let us take for an example the celebrated bull Shakespeare, said to have been the best of Longhorn bulls, as an individual and as a breeder. By referring to the diagram presented on the next page, which gives his extended pedigree, his breeding will appear at a glance. The Westmoreland bull was put to the first of the Canley heifers, known as Old Comely, and produced the bull Twopenny, a very widely esteemed bull. Twopenny was then put to his own dam and produced a heifer known as the "Dam of D," and also to the other of the two original Canley heifers, called the "Canley Cow," twice in succession, getting the "Son of Twopenny" and the "Daughter of Twopenny." Thereupon the Twopenny cow out of Old Come-

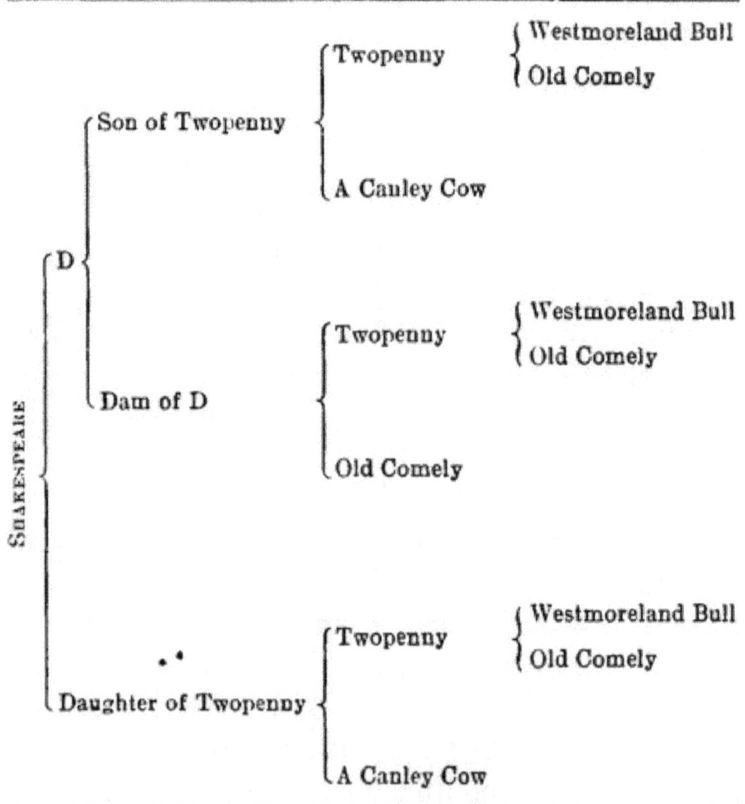

ly, being bred to the Son of Twopenny, produced the noted bull "D," and then "D," being bred to the "Daughter of Twopenny," produced Shakespeare. Of this latter bull, Marshall* says: "This bull is a striking specimen of what

* Marshall, "Midland Counties," quoted by Youatt.

naturalists term accidental varieties. Though bred in the manner that has been mentioned, he scarcely inherits a single point of the Longhorned breed, his horns excepted. * * * * His horns apart, he had every point of a Holderness or a Teeswater bull. Could his horns have been changed he would have passed in Yorkshire as an ordinary bull of either of those breeds. His two ends would have been thought tolerably good but his middle very deficient. He has raised the Longhorn breed to a degree of perfection which without so extraordinary a prodigy they might never have reached." This bull was very prepotent: "It was remarked," says Youatt, "that every cow and heifer of the Shakespeare blood could be recognized at first sight as a descendant of his." In the get of Shakespeare the highest point of excellence and reputation to which the Longhorn ever reached was attained. To quote Youatt once more: "What has become of Bakewell's improved Longhorn breed? A veil of mystery was thrown over most of his proceedings which not even his friend Mr. Marshall was disposed to raise. The principle on which he seemed to act, breeding so completely in and in, was a novel, a bold and a successful one. Some of the cattle to which we have referred were very extraordinary illustrations, not only of the harmlessness but the manifest advantage of such a system; but he had a large stock on which to work, and no one knew his occasional deviations from this rule, nor his skillful interpositions of remote affinities when he saw or apprehended danger. The truth of the matter is that the master spirits of that day had no sooner disappeared than the character of this breed began imperceptibly to change. It had acquired a delicacy of constitution inconsistent with common management and keep, and it began slowly but undeniably to deteriorate. Many of them had been bred to that degree of refinement that the propagation of the species was not always certain."

But the example had been taken to heart, and many breeders began to adopt with many kinds of stock the "Bakewell method." In the Short-horn counties a number of breeders began a general movement toward improvement. They began with the Bakewell method in a modified form, and perhaps never used it in so extreme a form as did some of the Longhorn breeders. The Collings, for instance, the most notable as improvers in the Short-horn field, did not use their great bull Hubback in anything like the incestuous manner that other bulls were used. It was not till Favorite (252) appeared that the great piece of in-and-in breeding in Short-horn history was inaugurated. Favorite's sire and dam were both by

Foljambe, so that he had a double cross of Hubback, but he was full of miscellaneous blood. Mr. Colling found him a remarkable sire and a bull of great vigor, and used him on his own get, and in a few cases bred him to his own calves out of his own calves. His wonderful powers gave a very satisfactory series of results, and to him trace a large portion of the most esteemed Short-horn families. After Mr. Colling's time the Favorite blood became so famous that in some cases the most extraordinary closeness of breeding was followed. Take for example Mr. Adkin's cow Charmer (E. H. B., Vol. VI, p. 295), calved in 1839, thirty years after Favorite's death. This cow traces in no less than four hundred and eight lines to Favorite, and as Foljambe and Hubback are each represented twice each time that Favorite occurs, to each of them at least eight hundred and sixteen times. I say at least, for she traces to each of these bulls many more times, especially Hubback, along other lines through Ben (70), Old Cherry, Lady Maynard, Broadhooks, and many others. I have not calculated the exact number of times that Hubback appears in the pedigree, but it is considerably over one thousand times. A number of Mr. Booth's cattle show an extraordinary interfusion of the Favorite blood. Take for example his celebrated bull Crown Prince (10087), which shows 1,055 lines to Favorite. This bull was crossed on Red Rose by Harbinger, which boasted no less than 1,344 lines of that highly-prized blood, so that the joint legacy to their offspring was 2,399 crosses from Favorite, and consequently they were more than 5,000 times descended from Hubback (4,798 through Favorite, the others through a variety of lines). But as these lines had been gathered up in a large number of generations and greatly intermixed, Mr. Carr ("History of Booth Short-horns") is justified in saying that "it will not do," in calculating the amount of in-and-in breeding practiced in this family, "to claim bulls as of kindred blood on this ground only."

It would be easy to quote a number of instances showing a tremendous number of lines centering in those early bulls. But from the beginning there were a very large number of breeders of the various sorts—the Holderness, the Teeswater, and other varieties of Short-horns—and the tendency, except with a few breeders, was to use the get of the celebrated bulls on great numbers of widely-drawn strains. The ever-widening circle, the early movement to exportation to foreign lands, effectually prevented the kind of concentration of blood secured in the improved Longhorn. I shall consider in a subsequent chapter the special cases of some of the more celebrated breeders who continued to follow in-and-in breeding for a long period of years. Were it necessary instances drawn from the early history of most of our improved breeds could be cited showing the predominant influence of one or two early bulls on the race history.

Nor has it been otherwise in the history of improvement in other animals. Some of the more fastidious breeders of the Thoroughbred race horse insist that every animal must trace in every line to an oriental source. As only comparatively few Arabs and Barbs were ever imported into England such pedigrees when fully extended would exhibit a great convergence as the further end was reached. Such a diagram would be very remarkable, as the theory on which the Thoroughbred has been all but universally bred is one of avoiding anything approaching close breeding, so that a rapid expansion of blood-lines followed the earlier and necessary close breeding. In many varieties of Bantam fowls in-and-in breeding has always been resorted to; indeed, it has been found almost impossible to maintain the very small size of these fowls where they are not constantly closely interbred. The same is true of many varieties of "toy" pigeons, the tiny size being maintained by the most constant return to a single line of blood—mating brother and sister, and similar cases of incestuous crosses.

Much experiment with many varieties of animals has given a few great facts that are very generally accepted; besides these, there are many significant facts the force and weight of which are greatly controverted. We must now examine into both of these classes, and if possible draw some practical conclusions from them.

It is conceded on every hand that the Bakewell school of breeders began on a correct principle. Given a large number of animals, only a few of which are possessed of certain desired qualities, we must take these few and interbreed them; select again from the offspring of these such as exhibit the desired qualities in the highest degree, and interbreed them, and so on till the whole number of produce shall show a general conformity to the type sought. A few generations are generally sufficient to fix the type; to fix it so as to make it capable of transmission to any ordinary stock of the unimproved sort with which it may be crossed. The question then arises, How far is such a course to be persisted in?

We have noted already the physical decay resulting from long-continued close breeding in the Longhorn. It is pretty well established that in-and-in breeding invariably results in general deterioration of the whole animal nature when long continued. Just what is the limit line has never been determined, and indeed can never be, for much depends on the vigor and vitality of the stocks used. It is well recognized that a breed with fresh blood, unpolluted by the evils so commonly resulting from the unnatural, artificial life of a domestic condition, will stand in-and-in breeding better and give more valuable results from such a system than a breed long domesticated and with a system impaired by long continuance under artificial conditions of life. The decay consequent upon such in-and-in breeding attacks first of all, in most cases, the generative organs, producing reduced fecundity, infertility, impotency, tendency to abortion, etc. These disorders are accompanied or followed by organic troubles affecting the animal in those organs which for any reason are weakest, most frequently appearing as pulmonary and tuberculous diseases, scrofula in all its many forms, ophthalmia, etc. The first appearance of these symptoms is not a danger signal. The danger was long ago; the damage is already done. Such forms of disease are strongly prepotent, and will linger long in the decayed stock upon which they have been engrafted.

Among human beings we are all familiar with the divine law which forbids incestuous marriages, and with the fact that this law has been engrafted into most human codes, and scarcely less with the cases of idiocy, insanity, consumption, and scrofula which have resulted from a defiance of this law, sometimes only in spirit, as by the frequent intermarriage of relations not within the limits of incest.

The force of the argument against in-and-in breeding has been sought to be broken by citing the case of the Jews. There is much to be said for this example. In the earliest record of the race we see in the marriages of Abraham and Sarah, of Isaac and Rebecca, of Jacob and Leah and Rachel that close and intimate intermarriage which in an early stage and under the circumstances presented by a primitive race dwelling near to a state of Nature is in accord with general experience the most potent influence for fixing a race type. But we see as the race is more expanded the stringent law against incest, and among a numerous people dwelling in a rough and mountainous country, and at no long period acquainted with the enervating influences of a luxurious life of ease and dissipation, such as was the state of the Jews until the destruction of Jerusalem by Titus; or dwelling in every land and among all peoples, separate and apart, communicating and intermarrying with their kindred in many lands, excluded from most of the temptations to luxury and vice by caste lines, as is their now long-existing condition—it would not be strange that, incest being strenuously inhibited, close racial affinities could long be maintained without impairing the power of the race. And yet granting all this, admitting the occasional greatness of Hebrews, their proverbial success in trade, the now rare physical beauty of the women, the Jew is not a dazzling argument in himself, as he now exists, for the practice of in-and-in breeding.

Next to the Jews the Egyptian royal line of the Ptolemies has done most service in the support of in-and-in breeding from a human standpoint, but Francis Galton, the able investigator of the phenomena of inheritance, handles the Ptolemy claim rather roughly in his work on "Hereditary Genius."* The first of the Ptolemies was the son of Philip II of Macedon by Arsinoe, and consequently a half-brother of Alexander the Great. Ptolemy Soter I "became the first king of Egypt after Alexander's death" and was highly rated by Alexander. "He had all the qualities of an able and judicious general. He was also given to literature and patronized learned men. He had twelve descendants who became kings of Egypt and who were called Ptolemy, and who nearly all resembled one another in features, in statesman-like ability, in love of letters and in their voluptuous dispositions. This race of Ptolemies

*"Hereditary Genius," pp. 150 to 153.

is at first sight exceedingly interesting on account of the extraordinary number of their close intermarriages. They were matched in-and-in like prize cattle, but these near marriages were unprolific; the inheritance mostly passed through other wives. Indicating the Ptolemies by numbers according to the order of their succession, II married his niece and afterward his sister; IV his sister; VI and VII were brothers and they both consecutively married the same sister; VII also subsequently married his niece; VIII married two of his own sisters consecutively; XII and XIII were brothers, and both consecutively married their sister, the famous Cleopatra. Thus there are no less than nine cases of close intermarriages distributed among the thirteen Ptolemies [nine generations only]. However, when we put them as below in the form of a genealogical tree we shall plainly see that the main line of descent was untouched by these marriages, except in the two cases of III and of VIII. The personal beauty and vigor of Cleopatra, the last of the race, cannot, therefore, be justly quoted in disproof of the evil effect of close breeding: on the contrary, the result of Ptolemaic experience was distinctly to show that intermarriages are followed by sterility."

Nor is this all that our learned author might have said. The ablest of the Ptolemies was undoubtedly Soter I, the first of them all, and next to him Philadelphus, whose mother was unrelated to his father. And the lovely and vigorous queen who brought this incestuous and ignoble line to a fitting close was barren when married to her brothers and only bore the sickly and short-lived Cæsarion, the child of Cæsar, in all her amours. Set over against this record that of the outbred members of the family. Philip II, of whom Cicero said in looking back over his career, that he was "always great" though cut off at the early age of forty-seven by a violent death, links Alexander, who died at thirty-two, and Ptolemy Soter I, his sons, and Pyrrhus, his cousin, one of the greatest generals and statesmen of antiquity, in a relationship of vigor and ability which makes the poor residuum of their noble blood to be found in the Ptolemies no better than the lees of the wine.

Outside of these notable cases, the verdict of humanity is against the intermarriage of near relations. I have seen in my own observation many cases in which it was unquestionably true that too close intermarriage had resulted in physical decay in the offspring. I have in mind at this moment as I write cases of idiocy, consumption, scrofula, diminished size and impaired vitality, infertility, and reduced, almost destroyed, fecundity, growing out of this cause. The voice of medical science and human intelligence is clearly at one in regarding close breeding, especially when so close as to be properly within the definition of in-and-in breeding, as highly mischievous.

But let us pass on to a department more nearly connected with the subject of our particular study. A very noteworthy case of an experiment with swine is recorded by Mr. John Wright, a leading writer on agricultural topics. Says he in the course of some remarks on inbreeding: "In pigs the writer's experience was considerable, inbreeding from three or four sows at the same time, all descended from the same parents, boar and sow; these were put to the same boar for seven descents or generations; the result was that in many instances they failed to breed, in others they bred few that lived; many of them were idiots—had not sense to suck, and when attempting to walk they could not go straight. The last two sows of the breed were sent to other boars and produced several litters of healthy pigs. In justice to the advocates of the in-and-in principle, it is but right to state that the best sow during the seven generations was one of the last descent. She was the only pig of that litter. She would not breed to her sire, but bred to a stranger in blood at the first trial. She possessed great substance and constitution and was a very superior animal." It would seem that this high character was secured at rather a high cost. The only pig of a litter to begin with; partly infertile—so much so that had not the in-and-in system been abandoned precipitately she would have been the last of her line; a barren sow in all practical senses; the one fine animal out of all that company of the dead-born, the impotent, the idiotic, the halt and infirm. Truly a costly beast to breed.

A recent writer in commenting on this case advances the following ingenious theory*: "That the procreative powers were not destroyed, but remained latent, is shown by the fact that the sows bred freely with the boars of another family. With boars of their own blood they could not be expected to breed, as the powers of fecundity in such case would be latent in both male and female; but when they were bred with animals in which the reproductive function was *not* latent the defect was corrected." Latent, or impaired almost to the degree of total destruction, the case most admirably illustrates the fact that Nature has placed a barrier beyond which in-and-in breeding cannot be carried. This case illustrates well some of the most important facts of in-and-in breeding. It shows absolutely the extreme tendency to physical and mental decay; it shows this

* Prof. Manly Miles in "Stock-Breeding," page 169.

tendency and it shows a large number of the forms which this tendency will take. For instance, decreased fecundity, impaired fertility, (the difference between these should be kept well in mind: the sow above named in her failure to breed to a related boar showed impaired fertility; her dam when she produced her, one pig at a litter, showed decreased fecundity) disease of the procreative organs in frequent births of dead young, transmission of weak organisms seen in the idiocy and incapacity of some of the young, and so on. Over against these things are set the case of an extraordinarily superior animal in form and appearance. These fine animals have been produced again and again by such a course, but nearly always at a cost analogous to that witnessed in the case of this sow.

We have perhaps had enough examples to see the theory and the experience of breeders in applying in-and-in breeding. It may be briefly summed up as follows:

The theory of in-and-in breeding rests first on the view that the way to obtain the best cattle is to select the best obtainable animals and breed them and their offspring together over and over again, thus maintaining their excellencies free from the intermixture of any less excellent blood, and making by constant interfusion the blood of all the animals identical and so preventing the appearance of any feature outside of the animals originally selected; and second, that the in-and-in bred animal is prepotent over any and every other.

This latter proposition has been questioned by some as only true when the animal has special vigor, though in the main it is probably approximately true.

While recognizing the force of the claims made for in-and-in breeding, some breeders have been alarmed at the physiological dangers besetting that course and have adopted a modified view of the general theory generally called "line breeding," a brief outline of which will now be given.

LINE BREEDING.

THERE has been much discussion as to what is meant exactly by "line breeding." It is comparatively new as a word applied to a distinct system of breeding, and it has acquired something of a special character, in addition to its old general application, on account of its adoption by certain breeders to describe their own peculiar methods. It may, perhaps, be not inaccurately defined as the process of breeding within a few closely related stocks or families, no animals being interbred which are not closely connected in the general lines of their blood, the idea being apparently that all the animals so interbred are of the same "line" of descent. This, if pressed to close accuracy, would, of course, be the same as in-and-in breeding. But by a little latitude of expression the "line" might be, and indeed has been, so expanded as to include relationships more distant than would properly be thought within the true purview of in-and-in breeding.

Historically this practice is an offshoot from the main stem of in-and-in breeding. It is now a number of decades since the last successful scientific breeder deserted the sinking ship of continuous in-and-in breeding. On the heels of that expiring system followed a practice which some of its exponents sought to distinctively designate as inbreeding, but this term was not sufficiently differentiated from in-and-in breeding (perhaps the practice described by the two terms were none too separable to the vulgar eye) to be generally understood as a different practice, and these men, as they grew more and more away from any general practice of incestuous breeding, took up the term line breeding as designating their method. The actual affinities of "line breeding" are beyond the power of human ingenuity to discover. The process of defining the term has been a perfect "open-entry," "go-as-you-please" contest, in which many have taken a part and nearly all have desired an exclusive liberty of action, ruling off all competitors. The reason of this is not far to seek.

Beginning with any given pair of animals if their produce be interbred and their produce again, and the progeny should be numerous, then after the third generation the crosses would cease to be incestuous, but would continue to be "line bred." Now this is exactly analogous to the case of the Jews, in which in-and-in breeding early gave way to line-breeding of this sort. As I understand the process, this is, properly and logically speaking, the only true definition of line breeding. But as this has been largely devised to fit actual cases much deviation has occurred. Some have taken their own herds at a given period and made that a starting point and counted all as line bred which showed no cross outside of the animals thus started with. A well-known instance of such a case is that of a number of breeders who bred exclusively from the seven families which were owned by Mr. Bates at the later period of his life, admitting also such outcrosses as Mr. Bates himself used on these families.

The idea is from a narrow standpoint to breed only to animals showing no cross outside of a single family; from a latitudinarian point of view the family may be represented by a dozen or more families, a whole herd or any other body. Perhaps to the uninitiated he who breeds only to such cattle as are admitted to the herd book would as properly be a line breeder if he chose to take that as a basis. But he would probably be quickly convinced of the fact that he was uninitiated. It is not included in the definition, but it is nevertheless true that the basis of a system of line breeding ought to be small enough to give the line breeder a "corner" in the stock. An unprolific family is thus the chosen ground of most line breeders. If the family become too prolific it would be soon out of all control. Its kinship to in-and-in breeding thus becomes more noticeable; indeed, it is perhaps not too much to say that it is a modified form of that practice, and that most of those who practice it are in more or less close sympathy with the theory of in-and-in breeding, and have only departed from it just so far as they were driven by the fears of physical decay.

The aim of line breeding, as has already been pointed out by implication, is to secure and maintain a high degree of identity of blood, the object being to obtain as nearly as possible exact uniformity in the herd. It is quite possible to attain a most perfect conformity of type in this way. Herds long bred on this principle become more and more reduced to a single type. I say reduced advisedly, and here lies one of the dangers of the method. A common type is not undesirable, indeed it is often highly desirable. But it is only desirable when it is a superior type and the cattle are elevated to it. Great improvement has only been attained by the adoption by some skillful breeder of some high ideal type and the use of every means in man's power to raise the stock bred to that type. We have seen that changed conditions of life, especially excessive increase of nutrition, sometimes inbreeding, as in the case of the Longhorn bull Shakespeare, would produce variations for the wide-awake breeder to seize and fix by every means in his power, and so bring his stock to a type of great evenness by raising them to this ideal standard. This can only be done by infinite labor and pains. Nature never stands still; her laws require progress or decay will ensue. So if man supinely contents himself with any already attained standard and lets the work of man go on simply in an effort to fix without improvement, deterioration is almost inevitably the consequence. Every fault will fix itself. Faults and defects in forms and organisms are nearly always more surely reproduced than good qualities. Cattle thus bred commonly show a deterioration in size and vigor most of all. If the lines are drawn very close and narrow the same faults as are to be found with in-and-in breeding, in a somewhat less degree, are observed; and last, but by no means least, when the processes of fixing the type and deteriorating the animals have gone forward long, judicious outcrosses do not rapidly overcome the inbred evils.

I know an instance under my own observation of a splendid herd of excellently bred cattle in which a system of close line breeding has after some twenty years of experiment, under the supervision of good judges of cattle, steadily fixed two most deplorable bad qualities on nearly every animal in the herd.

This method is often exceedingly tempting, and a little specious reasoning often makes the temptation irresistible. Given a fine herd to begin with and these well bred, and the owner often thinks that he would like to breed just these cattle and no others; that he would like to make of them a race of cattle of high reputation and out of them win for himself present and posthumous fame as a great breeder. Day dreams like these are easily conjured up and are the common joy of all times and all people. We have all heard the oriental story of the idle youth whose father died and left him a small sum of money with which he determined to make a mercantile venture, and invested the whole of it in glassware and took his place in the market with his wares. Seized with a sudden ambition to succeed in his new way of life he pictured to himself a rosy future as a successful merchant. He saw his little patrimony increase vastly through constant and rapid turning over. He saw himself ere long a merchant prince and at last even called to the high honor of marrying the Sultan's daughter. Then he thought how he would treat her, how scornfully, how disdainfully, and finally would spurn her from him as she embraced his knees seeking his favor. But the reverie became too real for his welfare. In the moment of his fancied pride he put his thought into action and threw out his foot as if to spurn the princess—really to strike the basket which contained the hopes of all his glorious future, and to overturn it with its fragile burden in a mass of splintered crystal on the ground. All might have come true if —the ever-fatal if; how often it intrudes itself into the affairs of men!

The work often goes on with the utmost success for a time and entices with such allurements as a taste of success is sure to hold out. The danger never lies in the beginning, but in the persisting in such a course.

It is sometimes argued with no little show of plausibility that the deterioration and physical decay incident to very close and long-continued line breeding does not result from the close breeding but from an accidental constant reproduction of a defective or diseased feature overlooked by the breeder. Hence that such cases are the result of the carelessness of the breeder in overlooking some such defect rather than in any actual positive injury coming from line breeding. But as all animals possess defects of one kind or another, close line breeding must tend to fix them ineradicably on the offspring. It becomes just as needful then to resort to fresh outcrosses to counteract this as it is under the view that close interbreeding of the same family for generations leads to a positive evil. It after all matters little whether one perishes of a negative or a positive evil.

A recent writer* would seem to make the lines so narrow as to claim an exclusive right for cattle in-and-in or line bred to the term "high bred." Says he: "High breeding implies a careful selection of breeding animals within the limits of a family with reference to a particular type and regardless of relationships. High-bred animals are not necessarily in-and-in bred, although from the system of selection practiced they must be closely bred to a greater or less extent." Surely there are many very high bred animals which have been bred otherwise than "within the limits of a family," and yet some writers and breeders would really seem to regard "close relationships"—I quote from the author just cited—as "the necessary incidents of their practice," although some admit that as to the early improvers "close breeding with them was but a means of improvement and not an end that was thought to be desirable in itself." Such a distinction, however true originally, can seldom be maintained long in practice, especially if that practice is common to a large number of men. It is very easy to mistake an incident or concom-

* Miles, "Stock-Breeding," p. 139.

itant for the efficient cause. And it is not to be denied that however much the early improvers were wanting in anything like a superstitious reverence for the fetich of close relationship, some who have come after them have not wanted a belief that positive virtue dwelt in and emanated from long-continued breeding within the limits of incest, or at least of a single family's lines.

How much the line theory is an outgrowth of the in-and-in breeding idea may be seen by a comparison of some early definitions of in-and-in breeding with that now most approved, viz.: that in-and-in breeding is breeding within the limits of what is known as incest in man; is, in fine, "incestuous breeding." Thus Youatt says that it is "the breeding from close affinities," which certainly embraces line breeding. "Johnson's Farmers' Cyclopedia" says it is the "breeding from close relations." Another writer defines it as "breeding from the same family, or putting animals of the nearest relationship together." All of these read more like definitions of line breeding than of in-and-in breeding.

Haply we have a most admirable illustration of this method furnished us on a large scale, and in a condition as little artificial and as near to a state of nature as possible in the white, so-called wild cattle of England, which are more truly half wild. A brief inquiry into their history, circumstances and condition, will be instructive in this connection, and I shall give a resumé closely following Mr. Darwin's account, of which the following is a close paraphrase where it is not verbally quoted:

Three forms or species of *Bos*, originally inhabitants of Europe, have been domesticated. *Bos primigenius* existed as a wild animal in Cæsar's time and is now semi-wild, though much degenerated in size in the park of Chillingham; the Chillingham cattle are less altered from the true primigenius type than any other known breed. The park is so ancient that it is referred to in a record of the year 1220. The cattle in their instincts and habits are truly wild. They are white, with the inside of the ears reddish brown, eyes rimmed with black, muzzles brown, hoofs black, and horns white, tipped with black. Within a period of thirty-three years about a dozen calves were born with "brown or blue spots upon the cheeks or necks; but these, together with any defective animals, were always destroyed." The wild white cattle in the Duke of Hamilton's park, where I have heard of the birth of a black calf, are said by Lord Tankerville to be inferior to those at Chillingham. The cattle kept until the year 1780 by the Duke of Queensbury, but now extinct, had their ears, muzzles, and orbit of the eyes black. Those which have existed from time immemorial at Chartley closely resemble the cattle at Chillingham, but are larger with some small difference in the color of the ears. "They frequently tend to become entirely black; and a singular superstition prevails in the vicinity that when a black calf is born some calamity impends over the noble house of Ferrers. All the black calves are destroyed." The cattle at Burton Constable in Yorkshire, now extinct, had ears, muzzle, and the tip of the tail black. Those at Gisburne, also in Yorkshire, are said by Bewick to have been sometimes without dark muzzles, with the inside alone of the ears brown; and they are elsewhere said to have been low in stature and hornless. The several above specified differences in the park cattle, slight though they be, are worth recording, as they show that animals living nearly in a state of nature and exposed to nearly uniform conditions if not allowed to roam freely and to cross with other herds do not keep as uniform as truly wild animals. For the preservation of a uniform character, even within the same park, a certain degree of selection — that is, the destruction of the dark-colored calves — is apparently necessary.

The cattle in all the parks are white, but from the occasional appearance of dark-colored calves it is extremely doubtful whether the aboriginal *Bos primigenius* was white. The primeval forest formerly extended across the whole country from Chillingham to Hamilton, and Sir Walter Scott used to maintain that the cattle still maintained in these two parks, at the two extremities of the forest, were remnants of its original inhabitants, and this view certainly seems probable.

These half-wild cattle, which have thus been kept in British parks probably for four or five hundred years, or even for a longer period, have been advanced by Culley and others as a case of long-continued interbreeding within the limits of the same herd without any consequent injury. With respect to the cattle at Chillingham the late Lord Tankerville owned that they were bad breeders. The agent, Mr. Hardy, estimates (in a letter to me [Mr. Darwin] dated May, 1861) that in the herd of about fifty the average number annually slaughtered, killed by fighting, and dying, is about ten, or one in five. As the herd is kept up to nearly the same average number the annual rate of increase must be likewise about one in five. The bulls, I may add, engage in furious battles, of which battles the present Lord Tankerville has given me a graphic description, so that there will always be vigorous selection of the most vigorous males. I procured in 1855 from Mr. D. Gardner, agent to the Duke of Hamilton, the following account of the wild cattle kept in the Duke's park in Lanarkshire, which is about two hundred acres in extent: The number of cattle varies from sixty-five to eighty, and the number annually killed (I presume by all causes) is from eight to ten, so that the annual rate of increase can hardly be more than one in six. Now in South America, where the herds are half-wild and therefore offer a nearly fair standard of comparison, according to Azara the natural increase of the cattle on an estancia is from one-third to one-fourth of the total number, or one in between three and four; and this no doubt applies to adult animals fit for consumption. Hence, the half-wild British cattle which have long interbred within the limits of the same herd are relatively far less fertile. Although in an unenclosed country like Paraguay there must be some crossing between the different herds, yet even there the inhabitants believe that the occasional introduction of animals from distant localities is necessary to prevent "degeneration in size and diminution of fertility." The decrease in size from ancient times in the Chillingham and Hamilton cattle must have been prodigious, for Prof. Rütimeyer has shown that they are almost certainly the descendants of the gigantic *Bos primigenius*. No doubt this decrease in size may be largely attributed to less favorable conditions of life; yet animals roaming over large parks and fed during severe winters can hardly be considered as placed under very unfavorable conditions.

Another close student of English cattle, Mr. H. H. Dixon, who contributed so many delightful articles to the press over the signature of "The Druid," gives some corroborative statements in regard to the Chillingham cattle in "Saddle and Sirloin." Among other things he says: "The steers weigh * * * from forty stone to fifty stone of fourteen pounds." That is from five hundred and sixty to seven hundred pounds, from which it is very plain that Mr. Darwin has not exaggerated the great deterioration in size. Prof. Miles, who is an advocate of close breeding, cites Mr. Darwin's account of the Chillingham cattle and says: "When I saw the herd in 1874 it numbered about sixty of all ages and sexes. Among them were several steers. The park-keeper informed me that they produced from ten to twelve calves annually, which agrees closely with Mr. Darwin's estimate [a little lower, it will be observed]. They are certainly not very prolific, yet the number of calves is, perhaps, as great as could be expected under the conditions in which they are placed. They exhibited no indications of degeneracy or lack of constitutional vigor, and I was assured that they were both healthy and hardy. After several hundred years of close breeding they are apparently as robust as animals that have frequently received infusions of 'new blood' by crossing."

We see that in the period between 1861 to 1874 there had been a slight decline in fecundity, and in the list Mr. Darwin gives he enumerates several which had recently existed but had become extinct. Not a great many years ago there were seven prominent herds of these well-known cattle, of which more than half have become extinct, one in very recent years, and only two show any vigor or prospect of long remaining as memorials of the distant past; and one of these, if I am not mistaken, is of the polled variety.

I think it is easy to read between the lines of all descriptions of these wild or half-wild cattle a warning against true and long-continued line breeding. The conditions under which they have lived would seem to be the most favorable as far as the individual goes for maintaining the physical strength and vigor. The dangers and vicissitudes of a wholly wild life are averted, and while protection and abundant food are given none of the more enervating influences of domesticated existence are introduced. Add to these the selection of the vigorous males, already mentioned in Mr. Darwin's account, and it is sufficiently obvious that the conditions of their life have been by no means unfavorable, and yet decline and extinction have followed. Is not the question whether it was or was not brought about by close line breeding forced upon us? The answer is as easy given as the question is asked, though many may not see the facts in the same light as I do.

NATURAL BREEDING.

We now come to what I call "natural breeding." I have so called it for want of a more accurate term wherewith to describe it. It has been called by some "outcrossing," by others "mixed breeding"; but both of these terms are far too narrow and inadequate for us to adopt. By natural breeding I mean breeding with the sole object of securing the best possible offspring. Outcrossing and mixed breeding alike fetter us to the idea of families and blood lines. We can only outcross when we have a family line to supply the "in" of which the "out" is the opposite idea. So we can only "mix" when we have some definite quantities to mix, as families, etc. In both of these terms an accident of the method pursued has been confounded with the essence and a name has resulted which is at once a misnomer and misleading.

The great central idea of the theory of natural breeding is that of selection—a selection akin to natural selection, whose outcome is the survival of the fittest, but akin to it in just the same way that instinct is akin to reason. Nature tends to preserve an average; so natural selection in all normal cases tends to maintain a dead level. Man, when he applies one of Nature's lessons, strives at once to eliminate all but those factors and influences which are above the average. Hence man's work tends always to destroy the average and results in raising it if intelligently applied, or lowering it if unwisely exerted. Instead of concentrating the mind on family lines the view becomes world-wide, one analogy won from Nature's laws being strictly followed up, namely, the close continuance within the bounds of the species or variety which we have chosen for our field.

Hence the great consideration is how to improve the breed, and the individual being the sole unit, how to improve the individual. The only road to the general improvement of the breed lies too plainly through special improvement of the individual to deserve discussion. Hence it is that "individual merit" may be said to be the great watchword of this method of natural breeding. We may therefore define natural breeding as that method which aims to produce the best animals by careful selection and interbreeding of the best obtainable animals.

That this idea is far broader than anything which can be defined as outcrossing or mixed breeding must be obvious to everyone. We shall see as we advance, however, in the discussion of the subject that the concepts represented by those terms form a part of the scheme of natural breeding. In fine, that outcrosses are the rule in natural breeding.

Two or three antecedent propositions are important to an intelligent comprehension of the aims of this method. In the first place it should be clearly understood that the great aim of breeding is to produce animals; secondly, animals of as high practical value for the actual uses of man's consumption as possible; thirdly, that where a standard of excellence has already been attained by earlier breeders and improvers this standard should be carefully maintained; and fourthly, that wherever and whenever it may be possible this standard should be advanced and the breed improved. These propositions, stated in a negative way, may be said to be: first, everything tending to impair the constitutions, and particularly the procreative organs, is to be avoided; secondly, the cattle are not to be bred for pedigree or to other purely artificial standards; thirdly, that neglect of the useful qualities already obtained in the cattle is ethically wrong, and to permit such qualities to be atrophied or decreased by non-use condemnable; and fourthly, that a man who breeds valuable varieties of stock should never forget that they are a trust committed to his charge and that a neglect of any opportunity to improve on them is to prove false to a high trust.

It needs no argument to convince any matter-of-fact man who has no preconceived hostile views that the way to obtain the best results is to seek, wherever they are to be found, the best individual animals. Were this not so then the whole idea embraced in the great law that like produces like would be a delusion. Nor is there any other method to be derived from that law.

There is nothing in this view at all antagonistic to the theory which maintains the advantage of in-and-in breeding under exceptional circumstances. If such a proceeding be demanded in order to fix a specially desirable quality this method of breeding would favor it. It advocates the choice of the best to be had. If these "best" are few they must be in-and-in bred till they are numerous enough to allow wider latitude. It does, indeed, hold that, in-and-in breeding being apparently contrary to the laws of physiology and injurious to the produce of animals so in-and-in bred, should never be indulged in except with the utmost caution, and never persisted in one moment longer than demanded by the special conditions of each case. Just as some poisons of the deadliest nature may be taken with impunity when administered in small quantities to the great benefit and advantage of the sick, so in-and-in breeding may be resorted to in order to produce a desired result which can only be so attained, but always under the exercise of the highest degree of care and the most watchful caution that like the cases of cumulative action of certain poisons a similar effect be not here produced.

The principal reason, then, why this method of breeding is one of constant and repeated outcrosses is not so much that there is thought to be any great virtue in an outcross as that close breeding is avoided because it threatens a positive evil. To avoid in-and-in breeding is to breed more or less out-and-out. But it must not be thought that this is the converse of the course sometimes advocated by extreme in-and-in breeding, namely: that an inbred animal, though never so bad, is yet preferable for breeding to animals of the same family line to a complete stranger in blood, however excellent. This makes a distinct virtue of the fact of the near relationship. Here there is no such idea. The fact that an animal is unrelated is chiefly negative. If he is bad shun him. The determining quantity is individual excellence. If the choice lies between a poor and unrelated animal and a superior and closely-related one, the latter should be selected. There are no fetiches in this method. The aim is excellence;

the law of Nature is that excellence can only spring from antecedent excellence; consequently we arrive at the rule of practice—that no inferior animal should ever be used. Shunning in-and-in breeding as a fertile cause of deterioration and decay, it must be clearly seen that the necessity which would compel the breeder to use an animal to breed from which was closely akin to the animals crossed with it must be stringent and inevitable.

Is there, then, no advantage of a positive kind to be derived from outcrosses? Certainly there is. What has already been said was for the purpose of showing that there was no such claim made for an outcross as has sometimes been made for an incross. But fresh foreign blood, if itself healthy and vigorous, means an access of vigor to a family. Why this is so is perhaps not susceptible of a very clear explanation. It is like many another fact in natural history—a fact of observation. Like prepotency and atavism, it is well established as a phenomenon the explanation of which we are as yet unacquainted with. The effect of a cross of very distant blood is sometimes very notable. Animals brought from distant lands and bred together often exhibit remarkable increase of vigor. Increased vigor has great practical value for the cattle-breeder, as some of its most notable manifestations are increased fecundity, prolonged life and period of production, improved flesh and milk-making powers, and often highly-marked prepotency.

A recent writer on the theory of breeding says, in summarizing his remarks on this subject: "There is no one point on which practical breeders, as well as scientists, are more perfectly agreed than that the ultimate tendency of breeding in-and-in is injurious; that when carried to excess it will always result in a loss of constitutional vigor in the produce; that while its tendency may be in the direction of fineness of texture, lightness of bone, smoothness, evenness, and polish, it is invariably at the expense of robustness, strength, vigor, and power. On the other hand, scientists, as well as practical breeders, with perhaps equal unanimity concur in the belief that a cross in the blood usually gives increased size and vigor to the produce, and that cross-breeding, or pairing of animals of distant varieties, usually results in increased fertility."

Mr. Darwin is very decided in his view that crosses of unrelated blood are in themselves of high value. He says, for example: "The gain in constitutional vigor derived from an occasional cross between individuals of the same variety, but belonging to distinct families, has not been so largely or so frequently discussed as have the evil effects of too close interbreeding; but the former point is the more important of the two, inasmuch as the evidence is more decisive. The evil results from close interbreeding are difficult to detect, for they accumulate slowly and differ much in degree with different species; while the good effects which almost invariably follow a cross are from the first manifest." And again Mr. Darwin says: "The benefit from a cross, even when there has not been any very close interbreeding, is almost invariably at once conspicuous. * * * That evil directly follows from any degree of close interbreeding has been denied by many persons, but rarely by any practical breeder; and never, so far as I know, by one who has largely bred animals which propagate their kind quickly. * * * Almost all men who have bred many kinds of animals, and have written on the subject, such as Sir J. Sebright, Andrew Knight, etc., have expressed the strongest conviction on the impossibility of long-continued close interbreeding. Those who have compiled books on agriculture and have associated much with breeders, such as the sagacious Youatt, Low, etc., have strongly declared their opinion to the same effect. Prosper Lucas, trusting largely to French authorities, has come to a similar conclusion. The distinguished German agriculturist Hermann von Nathusius, who has written the most able treatise on this subject which I have met with, concurs." And again he says, in summing up his observations on this subject: "Finally, when we consider the various facts now given which plainly show that good follows from crossing [the word is here used with reference to crossing families and also 'distinct varieties'], and less plainly that evil follows from close interbreeding, and when we bear in mind that throughout the whole organic world elaborate provision has been made for the occasional union of distinct individuals, the existence of a great law of Nature is, if not proved, at least rendered in the highest degree probable—namely, that the crossing of animals and plants which are not closely related to each other is highly beneficial, or even necessary, and that interbreeding prolonged during many generations is highly injurious."

In the course of a lengthy and able examination of this subject, and the facts illustrative of it, Mr. Darwin shows the tremendous influence of a cross in such directions as increased fruitfulness upon deeply inbred stock. In our present inquiry we are considering the case of a constant adherence to a system of outcrosses—of crosses chosen for merit simply and for the negative quality of non-relation—consequently the sudden and deep impression he alludes to is scarcely to be expected. The reason of this lies on the surface. No decay, no loss of constitutional vigor having occurred, there is no negative force to be overcome, no evil to be rectified. By careful selection the breed has been kept on the stretch, and generation by generation maintained by correct breeding and feeding up to the highest attainable standard. A bull of fresh blood put on a herd of cows so bred would not be a new element in a mass made up of a number of infusions of a single old strain, but every line would stand for blood as fresh as his own. Where cattle are long bred in a single locality, even in the most open way, there is a tendency to assume a local type, and here we have a good opportunity of witnessing the influence of a totally new cross. Thus an imported bull from England will sometimes infuse into our American stocks the same kind of new life which is aroused in closely-bred stocks by the introduction of a foreign strain.

I was much struck by a recent observation of this fact by a contemporary writer in England a few months ago. In the course of a discussion of the relative merits of English-bred and American-bred Short-horns he observed that in his judgment the American descendants of English stock had not so much deteriorated (as was maintained by another writer) from the ancestral standard as departed from it. He esteemed them quite as good beef cattle in all, or nearly all, respects, but he thought that the type was a very different one. Most of the cattle he had seen belonged to one family, or more properly, group of families, which had been so interbred as to be almost one. Almost everyone conversant with American Short-horns remembered that these animals were, and their descendants are, of a well-marked type, and that one in a measure peculiar to them; another and equally distinct type being cultivated by other breeders; and it also would have almost certainly struck this English critic as a departure from the English type. I should have described both of these and two or three well-marked English types of today, as well as the clearly-defined Aberdeen Scotch, not so much as departures from an archaic type as equally local special developments of that type. I am inclined to think that there are more points of resemblance in each of these types to the old parent form, and each would be measured more satisfactorily by the old standard than by that of any of its contemporary standards. This has simply resulted from the nearly inevitable bending to surroundings. It is under the rule of Nature harder to exactly maintain any given form than to do anything else. Progress or decline is the motto written on all artificially modified forms. So even in the struggle to simply hold what has been gained, new elements intrude and local modifications arise and become, often unconsciously, deeply set in the animal type.

Mark the close analogy of all of these instances to the gardener's experience in securing desirable variations in his plants: transplantation, rich soils, oft-repeated changes, frequent cross fertilization, temporary close fertilization when the desired variety is secured, then cross fertilization with a degree of frequency corresponding to the natural habit of the plant. The analogy is striking and the principle is probably universal.

A gentleman who was once a large cattle-breeder and always a strong advocate of in-and-in breeding in cattle, said to me recently that a cross of Cruickshank bulls on the Rose of Sharons was remarkably successful. It was very contrary to his natural view, but in perfect accord with the best experience of scientists and breeders. In a long acquaintance with cattle-breeding and familiarity with the methods pursued in many herds, I have seen much which has led me to a thorough persuasion that the correct system was to breed the best to the best, and to avoid close affinities. Close study of the results in the show-ring lead me to the conclusion that while an occasional animal of great merit is found to be the result of in-and-in breeding, that a large proportion of winners are descended from winners, particularly on the sire side, and mainly out of families of cattle bred in a promiscuous manner. It would be easy to run over the experience of a life-time and bring forth a great number of instances to confirm this position; but a great mass of illustration, as it cannot by the necessity of the case reach demonstration by mere weight of quantity, however great, is of no value, and I shall therefore only educe a few notable and representative examples. One of the most remarkable animals I ever owned or saw was Loudon Duchess 2d. Her career in the show-ring was extraordinary and almost without a reverse, although exhibited from the time she was a calf at many fairs, both in Kentucky and several other States, during which time she bred regularly and produced calves of the highest class in every instance, her second and third calves being the scarcely less distinguished show-yard winners Loudon Duchess 4th and Loudon Duke 6th, both of which were esteemed by some excellent judges as of superior excellence to their dam. Loudon Duchess 4th, indeed, triumphed over perhaps the finest ring of females I ever saw gotten together, consisting of fifty-six head, at the Bourbon Co. (Ky.) Fair in the autumn of 1870, when she was a yearling. These calves were by Muscatoon, a bull of National reputation for his individual merit, its recognition in the show-yard

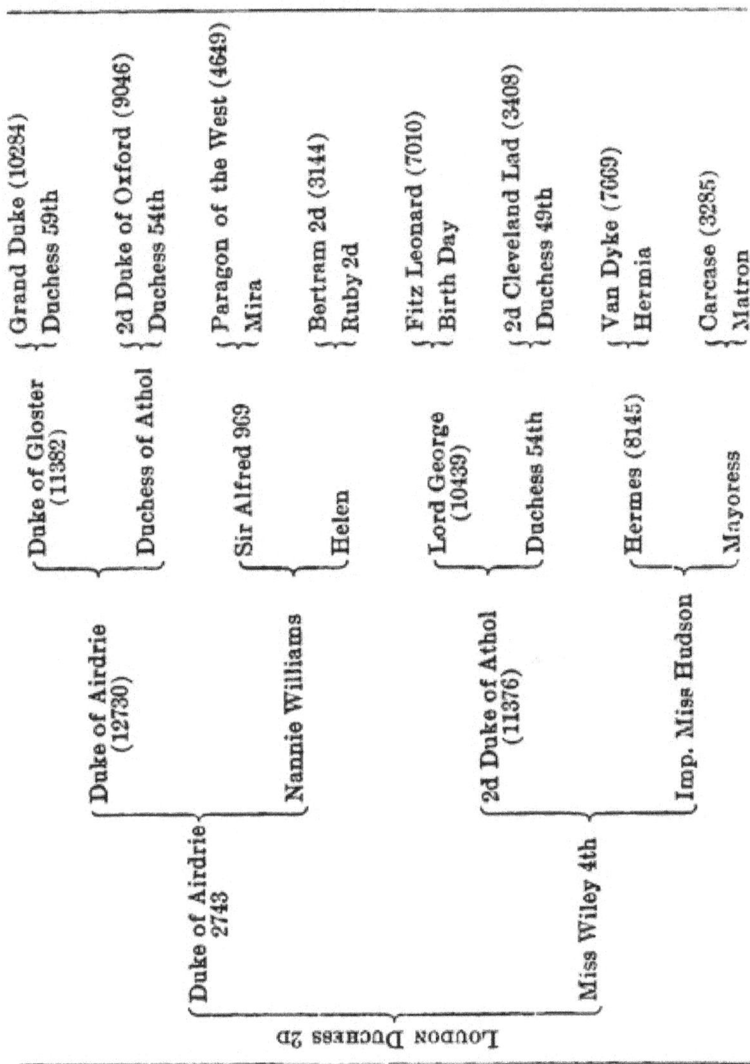

and his wonderful breeding qualities. If we examine the breeding of these animals we can but be struck by the very miscellaneous character of it. Turn to the extended pedigrees as displayed for a few crosses in diagrams

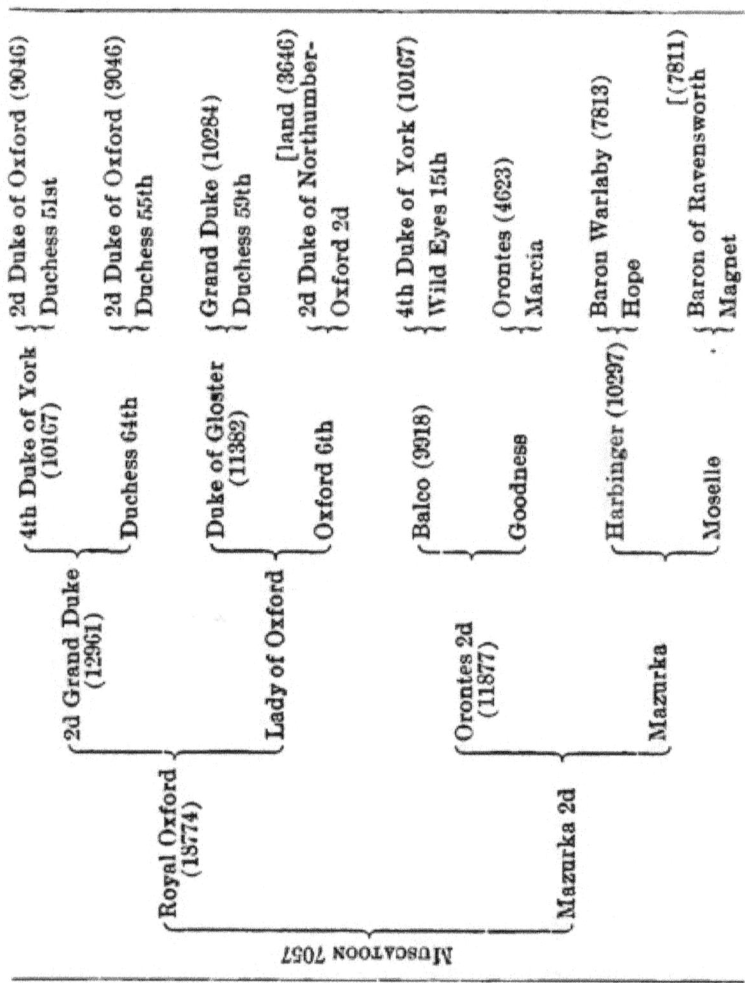

herewith and note first the mixed nature of each and the diversity of the one from the other. When interfused in their offspring the result is an increase of variety in the blood. Loudon Duchess 2d was also bred to Robert

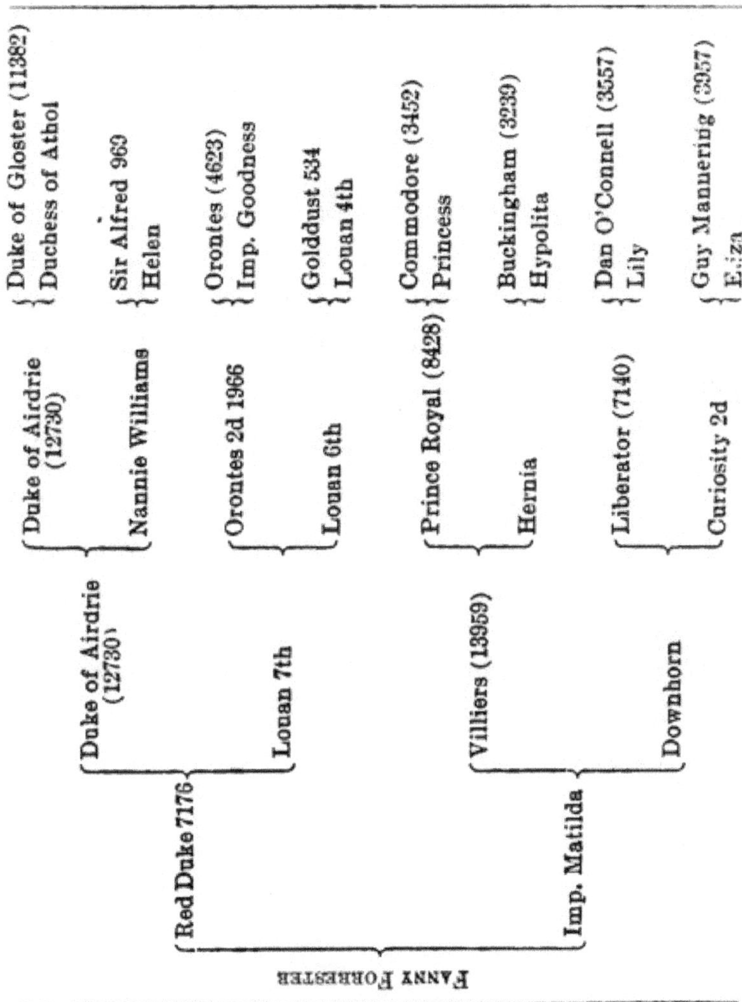

Napier (27310) with somewhat less success, but still she produced to him some unusually fine animals, and with his rich Booth breeding he

brought as great diversity to their offspring as did Muscatoon.

We find another notable example in Fanny Forester, one of the most superior animals that I ever saw, and looked upon wherever she went in a long and bright career as a show cow as a phenomenon of bovine beauty. She was as nearly perfect of her type, which was somewhat small, especially in contrast with some of the massive specimens of the Scotch breeders' handicraft now so much esteemed, as it was possible for her to be, and I believe met no serious rival in the show-yard of her own age except Loudon Duchess 4th. Her pedigree shows most miscellaneous breeding and a total neglect of any idea but getting good animals to breed together in the making of each successive cross.

It is of course impossible to reach any general rule from so slender a basis of particulars; nor was anything farther from my intention in citing them. They are, however, typical instances out of many that have come under my individual notice, and they may serve some good purpose as a counter-agent to the cases sometimes cited where a very fine beast has been produced by a system of in-and-in breeding. The narrow basis of generalizations of the boldest sorts upon single instances of close in-breeding is something only less surprising than the readiness with which such generalizations are received as logical and just inferences from the facts, and adopted as safe foundations for practice and experiment.

These cases are mere samples. It is not from them but from a careful and long-continued observation of the practice of many breeders, as well as my own long and wide experience, that I conclude that they are typical and are representative not merely of a class but of a large class, and that that class, while showing in itself varying degrees, exhibits at the same time a general unity, and is so large and so homogeneous as to almost unavoidably lead us to accept it as the ordinary case and to conclude that the tendency running through it is the rule; so that I do not think I am wide of the mark when I say that out of every ten celebrated prize-winners in recent years nine have been miscellaneously bred.

And it is further to be observed how prepotency runs with the vigor of the new blood which is introduced by outcrosses. One of the chief claims that have been made for the in-and-in method is the great influence that in-and-in bred cattle have in their prepotency over other cattle. But I have found that outbred cattle often show as high a degree of prepotency as those most deeply inbred. I have already instanced the case of Muscatoon, very

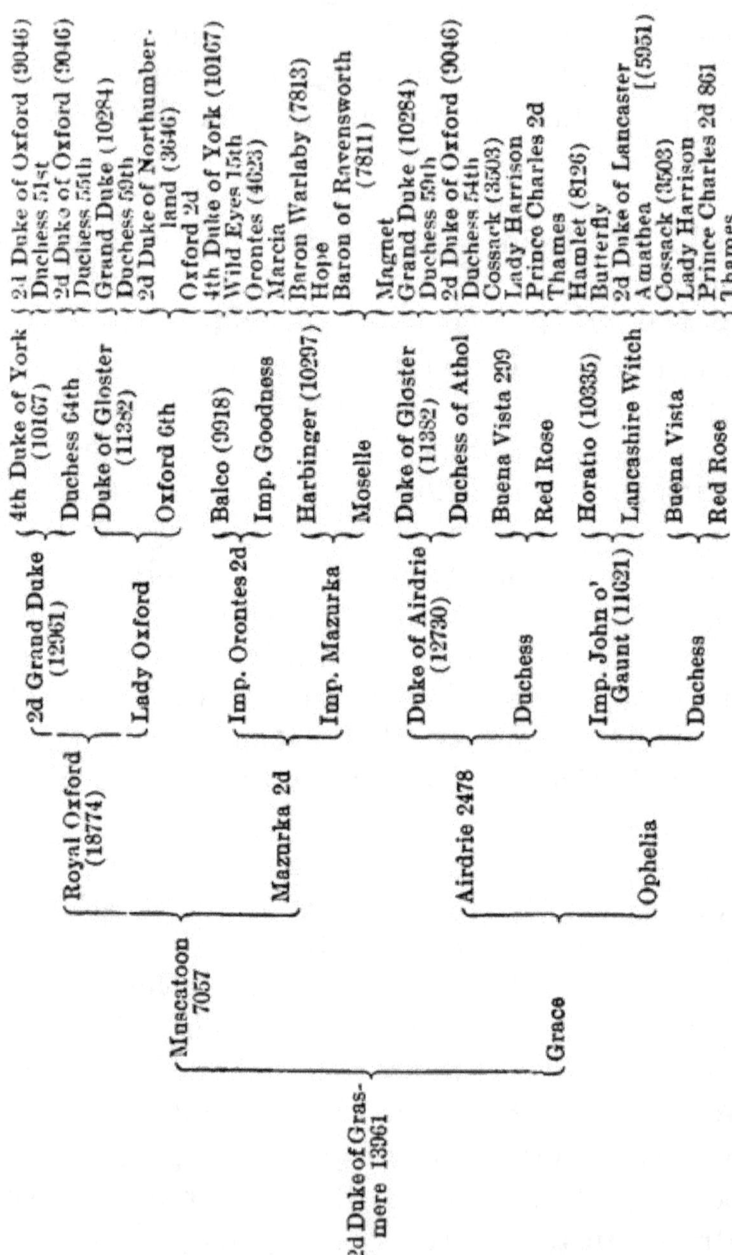

SIRE OF BARON BUTTERFLY 49871.

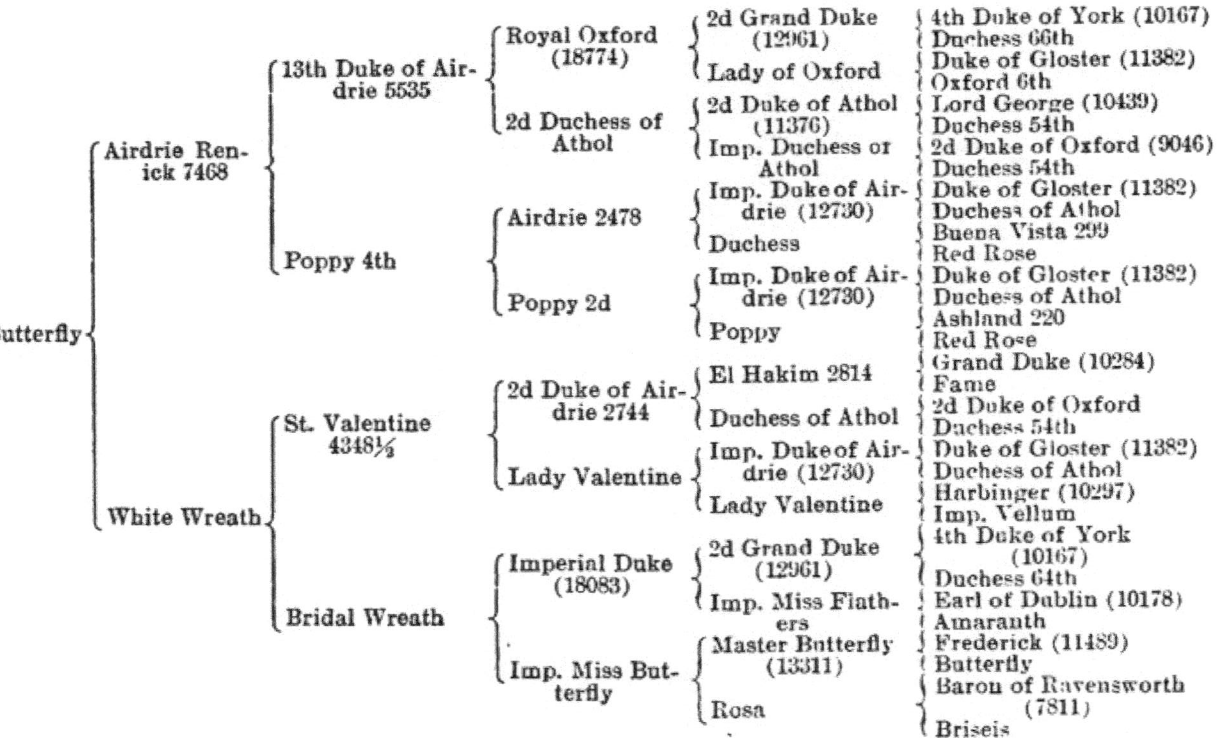

DAM OF BARON BUTTERFLY 49871.

nearly the greatest breeding bull I have ever known, and a great prize-winner. Another instance of the same qualities is to be found in Baron Butterfly, whose extended pedigree is also given. It will be noticed that in the 128 parts that may be seen from this diagram 38 are Duchess, 25 Oxford, 16 Booth, 5 Bates Red Rose, 1 Wild Eyes, 1 Belvedere, 9 Whitaker, 5 Princess, 4 Mason, 4 Barmpton Rose (the family from which he takes his family name), 2 Knightley, and the remaining 18 parts "scattering" among about as many families. This is surely pretty miscellaneous, as will be more fully realized by a glance at the extended pedigree. The same can be said of all the bulls spoken of in the chapter on prepotency as having exercised so great an influence in moulding my father's and my herd on account of their prepotency. Oliver, Goldfinder, Renick, Young Comet Halley, Cossack, as well as Muscatoon and Baron Butterfly, were full of variety in the families represented in them.

Among the bulls that have won very wide reputation of late years few have attracted so much attention as Mr. Cruickshank's celebrated sire Champion of England and Mr. Linton's Sir Arthur Ingram and Lord Irwin, and the miscellaneous character of their pedigrees is of the most obvious kind.

Even such breeders as had the most complete

faith in the in-and-in method have given expression to the opinion that unless in the hands of very careful and wise men there was much danger in long-continued close breeding. And it is certainly very plain that to the ordinary breeder who breeds cattle as a practical business, quite apart from any special fancy, regular breeding of strong, healthy stock, for which a demand at the full market price can be safely relied on, is the desirable course. A few men for fancy and fashion sake may prefer to breed animals uncertain and irregular as breeders, short-lived and delicate in constitution, producing many dead-born and sickly calves, for the sake of now and again one of extraordinary excellence which, perchance, may never produce a calf to perpetuate her own phenomenal excellence.

This method may therefore be safely commended as the safe course to all. From it the most satisfaction and most even results will be secured, and without any risk of doing injury to the breed of cattle which is cultivated. Those who desire to experiment and to breed for a fancy market, wholly dependent upon temporary and extremely evanescent fashions, may be trusted to find an agreeable road and to walk in it without very much regard to any one else's ideas or opinions, however well founded. But to the young and inexperienced, to the practical farmer, and the seeker for safe and plain methods, the system of natural breeding will continue in the future to hold the first place as it has in the past, supported as it is by the judgment of nearly all intelligent writers and all successful breeders, except a few whose life and self-interests were committed for special reasons to the other course. We will see in the next chapter what some of the great breeders have learned in regard to in-and-in and natural breeding.

HISTORICAL TESTIMONY ON BREEDING METHODS.

A DISCUSSION of broad, general principles, however widely illustrated, wants something of completeness, especially where the subject under consideration is one of immediate practical application. The individual propositions may stand out singly with clearness and force; but the question not unnaturally arises as to how they harmonize, and whether they unite and form a complete system. To be able, then, to give something like a connected account of the experience of some notable practitioners in any given sphere through a series of years will often throw a fullness of light upon the subject which cannot be obtained in any other way. That it is a difficult task to present in this way the life-work of any man or body of men is well recognized. It is necessary not merely to present the facts—the skeleton of the body of truth we essay to know—but to clothe them with the motives and purposes on the one hand, and the results on the other, which make the man's life-work a living, organic whole. Under any case the task is a difficult one. Where the facts, so far from being "so plain that he who runs may read," are controverted and denied, and the principles which may or may not have governed and controlled the actions, are the battle-ground of warring factions, then the task becomes ten times more difficult, and the most fair-minded and painstaking account is frequently assailed by partisans of one or both views. Yet these life stories are too valuable to be neglected. Experience has from immemorial days been one of the great guide-posts erected on the way through life—the experience, not only of each man for the better guidance of his own future, but of each man, also, for the aid of every other man who fares that way. What we can glean from the trials of other breeders in pursuit of the true method of breeding cannot but prove of value to us, then, and approaching it in the attitude of real seekers after truth we may, perchance, be vouchsafed a glimpse that may be of some value to all who would learn the lesson of their lives.

We have seen how Robert Bakewell struck out a new line in breeding methods, and with what notable success he met at the outset. His reputation was bruited abroad, and many enterprising men engaged in breeding various kinds of stock, following in his footsteps, began to make trial of his methods. Before Bakewell improved the Longhorns they appear to have been very generally regarded as distinctly inferior to the breed most commonly cultivated in Yorkshire and Durham which we know as the Short-horn or Durham, and which was then most commonly spoken of as the Teeswater or Holderness breed, from two of the localities in which it was largely bred. We have seen already that the celebrated Longhorn bull Shakespeare was described by a great admirer of that breed as very closely resembling an inferior Holderness bull. This breed—for, indeed, it seems to have possessed for many generations previous to this time a well-defined breed type—was bred with care and success by many men of the best character in the North of England, and was already highly valued for its qualities of beef and milk production, when, in the last decade of the eighteenth century, a number of breeders began to apply to them the Bakewell methods. Among these breeders the brothers Robert and Charles Colling have won the place of the greatest fame, owing to their active interest in the new methods, their confidence in themselves and in their cattle, their rare capacity for exploiting what they were doing, the real excellence of their results, and, perhaps quite as much as anything else, to the men into whose hands their cattle passed and who carried on most successfully the work of breeding, and not less that of exploitation in a manner and to a degree that would have refreshed the soul of Charles Colling could he have returned to these terrestrial scenes. Scarcely less able, and scarcely less successful were a number of others. Charles Colling seems to have regarded the cow Lady Maynard, which he purchased of Mr. Maynard of Eryholme, as unsurpassed by any product of his own long life as a breeder, but for our purpose the Collings stand out most strikingly; indeed they fairly accomplished more than all their contemporaries, and their just meed of praise is a large one. Shortly after the year 1780 they began to breed independently, having been raised under the shadow of the best of the old Short-horn traditions on their father's farm. They early adopted the Bakewell methods, and, Charles Colling having acquired Hubback, the corner-stone of the improved Short-horn breed was laid. The early days of the breeding of these brothers shows a cautious spirit; adhering, indeed, in a general way, to the Bakewell view, they were yet restrained by the older methods and the generally adopted physiological theory from throwing themselves too boldly into a course of close inbreeding. Consequently we find the Hubback stock inbred, but inbred with great circumspection and evident avoidance of extreme incrosses. It was not till the great bull Favorite (252) was produced by such a course of breeding that the whole Bakewell theory was put into operation. Favorite was inbred. His sire, Bolingbroke (86), and his dam, Phœnix, were half brother and sister on the sire's side, but more than this, both were descended from (the one being a daughter, the other a grandson) Lady Maynard, Mr. Colling's celebrated cow purchased of Mr. Maynard, who at the time of her sale called her Favorite, a name destined to become the special property of her famous grandson. The result of this was that Favorite had, like his sire and dam, one-half of the blood of Foljambe, and, also, he had three-eighths of the blood of Lady Maynard; that is to say, that seven-eighths of his blood were derived from these two sources. Of the blood of the great old bull Hubback he had only one-eighth, though twice descended from him through Foljambe in both instances. This was close inbreeding, but an analysis of Favorite's pedigree shows that the blood lines were very miscellaneous, and that no concentration of the blood lines of any particular animals had as yet been attempted. It is true that this bull is twice descended from the two most distinguished animals among his predecessors—Hubback and Lady Maynard—but Hubback in each case appears in the fourth generation, and the cross which produced Favorite was the signal, as it were, for the drawing together of the blood lines of the Maynard cow.

Hitherto the Short-horns seem to have been bred without any regard for pedigree in any way. They were indigenous, as it were, to that section of England, where they were bred, at least thoroughly fixed, as a natural element of the agricultural interests of that region, and bred for milk and beef, for the general farmer's purposes, for the dairy, and the butcher. They were in a state of ordinary domestication, unpampered, uninfluenced by any course of special breeding or improvement except such intelligent selection as the thrifty farmers had done to forward their profits out of the natural products of live stock. There was no danger of disease and want of stamina inherited from overbred ancestors and transmitted and transmissible through untold generations. The Collings had a task before them which was easy to point out, but difficult to perform. They had a sturdy, but somewhat rough, raw material; it was for them to cultivate and refine it. In Lady Maynard and Hubback they seem to have felt that Providence had given them exceptional specimens to work on. In Favorite, by a combination of these and other excellent specimens of the older, a later and modified starting point was obtained. In Favorite the new movement was begun. In short, it may almost be said that he was the embodiment of that movement. With him the

Bakewell theory was accepted and applied in its fullness in some cases in an extraordinary degree. The chosen stock was small. The interbreeding of the more successful results was necessary to maintain the excellence already gained. But it must be confessed that the Collings went farther than was demanded by this necessity, so much so that it seems clear that it was under a belief that close in-and-in breeding was in itself desirable. This idea was in some cases pressed to a great point, showing that while there was a conviction of the truth of the method embodied in it there was also a spirit of experiment closely connected with it, and a desire to see how far the course could be pursued with advantage and safety.

As far as can be gleaned from the rather meager accounts preserved to us Favorite was a bull of little above the ordinary merit, certainly not of phenomenal personal excellence. It was as a breeder that he was *facile princeps* among all the bulls of his day and generation. To him trace in one line or another almost every Short-horn family of any ancientness of lineage; indeed, there are few Short-horns which do not show in some line a cross to this old bull. He lived long and was used widely, but it was the depth of concentration to which his blood was carried that puts him in so notable a place. His great vigor and remarkable prepotency left a wonderful stamp. Take for example the celebrated bull Comet (155). He was by Favorite out of Young Phœnix, and she was out of Phœnix, the dam of Favorite, and herself by Favorite. This is an extreme example of incestuous breeding, and the result was regarded as a great triumph of the new method. Charles Colling said that he was the best bull he ever saw, and the general judgment of the day ratified this dictum, which is further confirmed by the enormous price he brought at the great sale of Oct. 19, 1810, which was 1,000 guineas (a little more than $5,000). At the time of the sale he was six years old, and a well-tried and highly-esteemed sire. In all respects he seems to have been a remarkable animal. He died of general decay, "breaking out into sores" all over his body, which seems to show that the course of in-and-in breeding had induced a scrofulous disorder, such as so often is caused by it. The bull North Star (458) was a full brother to Comet, and also a very fine bull, though not nearly so highly regarded as Comet.

In a number of the most notable bulls bred by the Collings the same extremely close in-and-in breeding is to be found. Thus the bull Lancaster (360), which brought the highest price, 621 guineas, at Mr. Robert Colling's sale of 1818, had a great deal of the Favorite blood, and also of the blood of Ben (70). He was by Wellington (680), out of Moss Rose by Favorite, out of Red Rose by Favorite, out of a cow by Ben (70), out of a cow by Foljambe, out of a cow by Hubback. His sire, Wellington (680), was by Comet (155), out of Wildair by Favorite, out of a cow by Ben (70), out of a cow by Hubback, etc. Lancaster (360) is described as "a white bull of fine quality, but narrow, thin, lanky, and small"; and it is said that during his life "a rumor was current that Lancaster was delicate." This, however, was denied, and he seems to have been a fine breeder.

The period of Robert Colling's active breeding is embraced between 1783, when he and his brother began to breed, and 1818, when he sold the greater part of his herd, only reserving those not in a condition to be sold. The animals reserved—eleven cows and their produce—were brought under the hammer in 1820, and from that date we count the final retirement of the Collings from the ranks of Short-horn breeders. Charles Colling had years before, in 1810, closed out his herd in a great sale and retired. During all this period they seem to have been consistent followers of Bakewell. We know that Robert Colling was personally very intimate with the elder improver, and for many years was more successful as a breeder of Bakewell's improved breed of Leicestershire sheep even than he was of Short-horn cattle. Says an English writer in speaking of Robert Colling: "There is little doubt that Bakewell's great principle of in-and-in breeding was carried out most successfully by the Collings. Father to daughter and mother to son were the principal direct alliances, and the system was continued so long as robustness and form were upheld." The Collings, indeed, may be said to have carried out the Bakewell method of in-and-in breeding to its utmost limit; to have found what advantages it really possessed, and to have proved that it could not be carried beyond a certain point. It was freely said that the cause of the Collings retiring was their having reached a point beyond which they could not advance, and that they found their stock becoming diseased and tending to retrograde. If this was so, the neighboring breeders had not lost confidence in their cattle, for they bid them in at good round prices. It is interesting to note that at Charles Colling's sale no family made such phenomenal prices as those having the "alloy," or Galloway cross. This outcross from the breed to another breed was a remarkable thing to do, and Colling had mingled the stream through grandson of Bolingbroke with his most esteemed blood. It was by some long claimed that Charles Colling distinctly regarded them as his best stock. The blood percolated very widely and got into most good herds without doing any damage that was ever heard of. Mr. Allen, in his history of Short-horn cattle, seeks to explain away the very remarkable prices the "alloy" cattle brought by saying that they were "high in flesh and most of them sold to the newer breeders, who were taken by the good looks of the animals," and seems to think this is a sufficient explanation of their high prices. But when one counts among the purchasers Messrs. R. Colling, Charles Wright, Thomas Booth, and Maj. Rudd and Sir Henry Vane Tempest, one-half of the explanation falls to the ground; and as it was to gain "flesh" and "fine looks" that the cross was made, if made for any purpose, the other half falls, too. As a matter of fact the Colling bulls had made a great family on the basis of the out-and-out Galloway blood with its North Country hardiness.

The Collings tried both plans, wavered somewhat at times, made the Galloway cross, and sent it into the herds of the best of later breeders, including Booth and Bates. But their legacy to the world was a belief in in-and-in breeding for the bulls, which they showed were never used at better advantage than when used on outbred or short-pedigreed cows. Not a few leading breeders, while seeking the blood of their great bulls Favorite, Comet, Lancaster, Ben, Albion, Pilot, and the rest, doubted the advantage of very close in-and-in breeding, and did not follow them. These were the great majority of breeders, and we could cite them with value, but it is better to study only those most apparently given to in-and-in breeding. Let us take Mr. Bates next.

Mr. Bates is often spoken of as the chief teacher by act and precept of the theory of in-and-in breeding, and even more has he been made the patron saint of the advocates of "line breeding." Mr. Bates was well acquainted with the theory and practice of in-and-in breeding, but no one need be told that of the modern invention called "line breeding" he knew nothing. He was no warm advocate of in-and-in breeding under any circumstances. Under any other than the most favorable conditions he openly declared his disapproval of it. He was, indeed, driven to practice it to no small extent, but this is explicable on other grounds than a belief in the wisdom of the procedure, and cannot be taken as contradicting his explicit declaration. Enamored of the excellence of his own cattle, and looking upon all else with a not very unprejudiced eye, he sought again and again to avoid diluting their perfection with blood which he regarded as very inferior to theirs, and thus strove to confine himself as closely as possible to his own stock. It is impossible on the one hand to resist the conclusion that the views of the line breeders of today would have received scant consideration at the hands of Mr. Bates; and on the other that he engaged in in-and-in breeding, whenever he practiced it, not as a thing good in itself, but as a necessary evil—an evil threatening harm—but rendered necessary by the supposed fact that no cross fit for his "pinks of perfection" could be found. Mr. Bell plainly sets forth in his so-called "History" what Mr. Bates' opinion in this matter was: "As to in-and-in breeding," says he,* "I believe that Mr. Bates considered that it required the greatest judgment and experience. He had the difficulty of obtaining bulls of as good or superior blood to his cows." Mr. Bell is not always as clear in his statements as he might be, nor is he invariably so reliable as not to be advantaged by a corroboration from another source. It is, therefore, well to cite another testimony to the same effect. This we find in a paper by Mr. W. Wood in the "Gardener's Chronicle" for 1855, and in another similar paper in 1860. He says that Mr. Bates expressed himself as thinking that "to breed in-and-in from a bad stock was ruin and devastation, yet the same might be safely practiced *within certain limits* when the parents so related were descended from

* Page 201.

first-class animals." "Undoubtedly," adds Mr. Bell, "many Short-horn cattle, by in-and-in breeding and high feeding and training, did become diseased." It is sufficiently evident from these statements that Mr. Bates did not regard the choosing of an animal of close relationship a universal recipe for good calves, but on the contrary as a dangerous thing to try; that he thought such a choice might be made "within certain limits," provided great care and judgment were exercised in the choice. The elements of such a choice, too, are not a few; the bulls chosen to make the cross must be "descended from first-class animals," and the cows not less so; bulls, too, of "as good or superior blood" with the cows which were unrelated to them must be attainable. Unless these conditions are fulfilled the promised end is "ruin and devastation." Truly this is far enough from a belief that there was any benefit to be gained by the mere act of inbreeding, or from any idea that there dwelt in "concentration of blood" some mystic and mysterious spell which worked a marvel in the produce. Mr. Bates was undoubtedly a man of prejudices, but he was a true and successful thinker and breeder, and he looked fairly and squarely at the problems with which he had to deal, and dealt with them honestly if with varying success.

Having thus cursorily inquired into the opinions expressed by this eminent breeder, let us now proceed to inquire into his practice. Mr. Darwin, who was certainly in this matter an unprejudiced student, sums up his examination into the method pursued by Mr. Bates as follows: "For thirteen years he bred most closely in-and-in, but during the next seventeen years, though he had the most exalted notion of the value of his own stock, he thrice infused fresh blood into his herd. It is said he did this not to improve the form of his animals, but on account of their lessened fertility."* As a general statement this may be taken as fairly indicating the general tenor of Mr. Bates' course. With this qualification, however, that even in the first thirteen years of close inbreeding there were two outcrosses quite extensively introduced, through the bulls Marske and 2d Hubback, though the latter was only half out and failed to restore the herd to its proper stamina and vigor. Mr. Dixon, indeed, says† that 2d Hubback was a distinct injury to the herd; but "it was only when Mr. Bates found that he had lost twenty-eight calves in one year, and solely through lack of constitution," that he was willing to give him up. Bell, however, does not agree with this view, and thinks

---

* "Animals and Plants Under Domestication," Vol. I, p. 147.

† "Saddle and Sirloin," p. 152, note.

that the loss of the calves, which certainly occurred, was not due to 2d Hubback. Whether the calves of 1831 died from some cause directly traceable to 2d Hubback, to general want of constitution, or what cause soever, Mr. Bates had used this bull in the hope of restoring strength and fertility to his cattle, and had failed. The cause of this failure seems most likely to have been the fact that he was not sufficiently outbred to effect the requisite revivification of blood, and to undo the evil which had been wrought. Mr. Lewis F. Allen, one of Mr. Bates' warmest admirers, sums up in his "History of Short-horn Cattle" Mr. Bates' experience up to this time as follows: "With the production of Duchess 32d (in 1831) Mr. Bates halted, and wisely. From the possession of his Duchess 1st in 1810, for a period of twenty-two years we find but thirty-one of her female descendants recorded in the herd book. There were meanwhile sundry bulls dropped from them, but mostly sold to other breeders, excepting those which he had used in breeding, and even they had been during some seasons let out for service to various parties. The simple fact was the Duchess cows, as a whole, had not been prolific or constant breeders, through abortions or other causes, and whenever they passed a year or two without breeding he fed off and slaughtered them."

If we analyze the results attained with this most celebrated family during this period we will feel no surprise that Mr. Bates should have paused and deeply considered the situation, and finally concluded that it was high time to make a radical change in his methods. He had begun with Duchess 1st, purchased of Mr. Charles Colling, a cow full of the blood of Favorite, and he at once began a system of inbreeding. Duchesses 2d and 3d were by Ketton (709), Duchesses 4th and 5th by Ketton 2d (710), and Duchess 6th by Ketton 3d (349). It would appear that already the necessity for new blood was seen, for Duchesses 7th, 8th, and 9th were by Marske (418), purchased at the Ketton sale, and Duchess 11th was by Young Marske (419). Duchess 10th was by Cleveland, and Duchesses 12th to 16th, inclusive, by The Earl (646), and the 17th by 3d Earl (1514), thus making a return to inbreeding. In like manner the 20th and 22d were by 2d Earl (1511). The half outcross of 2d Hubback is first to be seen in the 18th and 19th Duchesses, and then, indicating the strong sense of the necessity of a cessation of direct inbreeding, follow Duchesses 24th to 32d solidly by 2d Hubback. But the half measure was not enough. We have already seen that twenty-eight of the calves of 1831 died that year, and 2d Hubback was nearly related to the rest of the herd as well as to the

Duchesses. A complete bold break alone could save the herd; at least so seemed Mr. Bates to think. The suddenness and completeness of the change is well illustrated by the fact that the Duchesses from 33d to 43d—covering a period of seven full years—are everyone by sires having no drop of Duchess blood in them. Then, as we shall see that Mr. Richard Booth did under similar circumstances, he began to inbreed again the cattle which he had by this outcrossing filled with fresh and vigorous blood, but never again with the same recklessness that he had formerly shown. With the 51st Duchess the Oxford cross first comes in, that is in 1840; with the 52d, in 1841, the Holker cross first appears, and so on with constant admixture of strains till the last Bates Duchess—the 64th—was calved in 1849. When viewed in tabular form the marked changes in the method of breeding practiced on this family is very striking and instructive. Duchesses 1st to 6th are inbred; then 7th to 9th introduce the Marske cross; 10th to 23d are mostly inbred again, with the half outcross of 2d Hubback coming in occasionally, while it appears solidly from 24th to 32d; 33d to 43d are totally outbred, and from 44th to 64th are very carefully, even timidly, inbred and mixed. The practice of Mr. Bates clearly represents not merely the opinions expressed by Mr. Bates and quoted above but also the growth of those opinions, and in the last period we have a striking illustration of the conflict between his fear of too close inbreeding and his settled prejudice in favor of his own stock and unwillingness to introduce any other blood.

An examination into the motives which actuated Mr. Bates in his change of policy in 1831 reveals the fact that he was not half as anxious to obtain any particular strain of blood as he was to get some new and fresh strain of blood to cross into his stock. Mr. Dixon very accurately expresses it in the phrase which he employs. He says that Mr. Bates "began to cast about," and that very anxiously. He applied, but applied in vain, for Mr. Whitaker's Frederick (1060). He then sought Bertram (1716), but he was already sold to Col. Powell of Philadelphia to go to America. He would have been glad to get Norfolk (2377), and failing to obtain him sent cows to him. He used Gambier (2046), who got Duchess 35th. At last, after all this "casting about," he made a ten strike in obtaining the bull Belvedere (1706). Belvedere got Duchesses 32d, 33d, 36th, 37th, and from 39th to 43d. We have seen that Duchess 35th was by Gambier. Norfolk got Duchess 38th, while Bertram got Duke of Cleveland (1937), out of Duchess 26th. After a time the extremely strong outcross of the Oxfords was used, and when the bull Holker was used through him a return was made to the blood of 2d Hubback, which was now become an outcross owing to the outcrosses used between 2d Hubback and this descendant of his. Then, too, there was the Young Alicia cross in Lord Barrington (9308), the sire of Duchess 58th. It is evident that Mr. Bates never permitted himself to fall back into the error of his early breeding, but under the dominant influence of his superlative appreciation of his own stock used them as exclusively as he dared, and warily and tentatively mixed and mingled his strains of blood from 1838 to the close of his career as a breeder in 1849. The view expressed by Mr. Darwin, heretofore assented to in a general way, might advantageously be modified to some such statement as the following: Mr. Bates' breeding falls into three periods. The first, from 1810 to 1831, covering about twenty-one years, was his period of tutelage, in which he was largely governed by the theories then dominant, and in which he was engaged in making trial of those theories. This period is characterized by deep inbreeding in its early years, and in its later years by insufficient recoil from it. The second period, from 1831 to 1838—the period of his greatest independence of action—was one of strong and varied outbreeding, and during these years he made his herd capable of gathering the laurels which were to give it such lasting fame. The third period, from 1838 to 1849, was one of cautious mixture of in-and out-breeding—a time in which the herd lines were drawn as closely as seemed safe, in order to enhance their repute and value. Throughout this period Mr. Bates presents the aspect of one struggling against his prejudices and struggling in vain. It is important to notice that it was not till the close inbreeding of the first period had given way to different counsels that Mr. Bates began to win his fame as a breeder and his triumphs in the show-yard. His great show-yard triumphs followed upon the heels of his second period, that of outbreeding. It was in 1839 that, with the Duke of Northumberland, the Oxford cow, and the two Duchess heifers, he made his first great show, and it was in the following year that he clinched that victory with another, when the Cambridge cow and calf and the Cleveland Lad bull were brought forward. These victories followed on the heels of his outcrosses and give their results. This is not merely the clear inference from the facts before us; it is also Mr. Bates' own avowed opinion, for he declared: "My best stock are descended from 2d Hubback's daughters put to Belvedere, a union that has answered most admirably."* In other words, these two crosses,

* "Bell's History," p. 81.

one half out and the other a strong outcross, following one upon the other, produced his best stock. It thus appears from Mr. Bates' own testimony that it was the outcrossing which gave his herd its great excellence. Afterward careful inbreeding of outcrossed strains continued the excellence for a time, though fresh blood again (in the Oxfords) was soon demanded.

We have already noticed the conclusion reached by the great German student Nathusius, that no breeder of note ever followed inbreeding throughout life. This we see is true of Mr. Bates in a marked degree. He began with close in-and-in breeding, which he was compelled to abandon both in practice and theory and never returned to it. The Duchesses have here been used as the exemplar of his whole career because they were the pivot of his life as a breeder. What we read in them may be read in all.

Contemporary with Mr. Bates, and not less notable than he, both as men and breeders, were the Booths, Thomas and his sons Richard and John. The foundation of the great Booth herd dates as far back as the year 1790, about which time Thomas Booth began to actively breed the improved Short-horns. As descendants of the elder Booths still breed this noble breed at the old seats and still maintain the ancient strains in high excellence, the Booth name claims a place of extraordinary prominence in Short-horn annals. The sands of a century of continued labor in this one field are almost run, and the results of that long period are incalculable. This at least may be said, without overpraise, that the work which the Booths have done claims a higher praise when measured by its excellence than when measured by its quantity and the length of time in which it has been in progress. Thus, to quote only a single example of the estimation in which Booth cattle have been held, Mr. Dixon says that "Old breeders tell us that the sight of the Young Albion cows at Studley, in Mr. Richard Booth's day, is one of which they have never seen the equal."

The practical beginning of Mr. Thos. Booth's career in 1790 was the hiring of the bulls Ben (70) and Twin Brother to Ben (660) from Mr. Robert Colling. These bulls were by Punch (531), he by Mr. Robert Colling's bull Broken Horn, and out of a cow by the same bull; their dam was a Foljambe cow out of a Hubback cow. Thus he put himself in the direct line of the Colling movement of improvement—a line which he continued to pursue. Previous to 1790 Mr. Booth had owned and bred some of the old-fashioned Teeswater cattle; in other words, the so-called native or unimproved

Short-horns. He obtained one notable family from a Mr. Broader of Fairholme, a dairy farmer whose stock are said to have been "unusually fine cattle for that period—good dairy cows, and great grazers when dry, * * * of very robust constitution." Three cows purchased from this herd, "Strawberry Fairholme, Hazel Fairholme, and Eight-and-Twenty-Shilling Fairholme, have the honor of being the ancestresses of several illustrious families of Short-horns." This is a specimen of the kind of foundations the Booths sought, and it in no small degree explains their success. These sturdy, unimpaired stocks gave a fund of vigor calculated to resist much inbreeding. We find another example in the foundation cow of the great family generally known as the Isabella tribe, of which we are told* that "In the first year of his residence at Studley [1814] Mr. R. Booth bought in Darlington market the first of what was afterward known as the Isabella tribe. She was a roan cow by Mr. Burrell's Bull of Burdon, and, for a market cow, had a remarkably ample development of the fore quarters. She was put to Agamemnon. The offspring was White Cow, which, crossed by Pilot, produced the matchless Isabella, so long remembered in show-field annals, and to this day quoted as a perfect specimen of her

*Carr's "History of Booth Short-horns," p. 14.

race. * * * Isabella was the Rev. Henry Berry's [no mean judge] *beau ideal* of a Short-horn. * * * Isabella and her descendants brought the massive, yet exquisitely moulded fore quarters into the herd, and also that straight under line of the belly for which the Warlaby animals are remarkable. That such a cow should have had but three crosses of blood is striking evidence of the impressive efficacy of these early bulls, and confirms Mr. R. Booth's opinion that four crosses of really first-rate bulls of sterling blood upon a good market cow of the ordinary Short-horn breed should suffice for the production of animals with all the characteristics of the high caste Short-horn." The Darlington cow was sold to the master of a boarding school, eventually, as a milch cow, and she left behind her there a lasting memory for the "brimming pails of milk she gave." Mr. Booth's confidence in the effect of a few crosses on fresh, vigorous, outbred stock led to many more noble animals and notable families besides those sprung from the Fair-holme and Darlington cows. There is many a show-yard record which reveals how hard certain short-pedigreed Booth cattle were to beat. Perhaps it is permissible to think that the fresh blood of the cows was as potent a factor in the product as the concentrated blood of the sires. But this digression has already proceeded too far.

Mr. Carr says of Thos. Booth that he was no servile imitator. "He was a contemporary of the Collings, and began his career quite independently of them as an improver of the cattle of the same district, and he commenced it nearly at the same time. * * * He afterward did what wisdom dictated—availed himself of the Collings' best blood and incorporated it with his own. * * * Having judiciously selected the best animals procurable of both sexes, Mr. Thomas Booth was careful to pair such, and such only, of the produce of these unions as presented in a satisfactory degree the desired characteristics with animals possessing them in equal or greater measure, and unsparingly to reject, especially from his male stock, all such as were not up to the required standard. Having by these means succeeded in developing and establishing in his herd a definite and uniform character, he sought to insure its perpetuation by breeding from rather close affinities as in his opinion the only security for the unfailing transmission, and transmission in an increased ratio, of these acquired distinctions to the offspring. In tracing the pedigrees of these herds it will be seen that from the earliest period the same system of breeding from close relations which was pursued by the Collings was followed by the Booths."

In this passage Mr. Carr confused terms, or,

which is less probable, declares Mr. Booth's theory and practice to have been opposed. He says that Mr. Booth sought to perpetuate the excellence of his cattle "by breeding from rather close *affinities*," and then in the next sentence says that the Colling system of breeding from "close relations" was followed by the Booths. Doubtless he intended to say "relations" in both places. If this is so it may represent what the Booth theory was; certainly it represents what Mr. Carr believed to be the Booth theory. That the Booth practice varied far, even very far, from it, it will be easy to show.

In the first place new blood was constantly introduced into the Booth herds from many sources, chiefly market cows of the sturdiest type. In the second place constant and frequent resort was had to outcrosses, especially in that earlier time when the father and sons, Richard and John Booth, represented the family. In more recent times, which are too recent for our purpose at present, it is well known that disease has terribly injured these historic herds; that some of the more serious effects of in-and-in breeding have been felt in them, and that wholesale drafts from outside herds have been resorted to in order to maintain the actual and historic excellence of their grand families of cattle. We shall only dwell on some of the outcrosses introduced, and on them but briefly.

The first twenty years of Mr. Booth's breeding, down to the acquisition of Albion (14) at Mr. Charles Colling's sale in 1810, Mr. Booth had been pursuing the Bakewell method with frequent resort to very close in-and-in crosses, but with equally frequent resort to outcrosses, and he mixed all sorts of blood with the blood of Ben and Twin Brother to Ben, on which the herd in a certain sense was founded. A more miscellaneous collection of crosses than Mr. Booth's herd contained at the end of this time it would be hard to conceive of. It was a course of inbreeding with strong outcrosses at frequent intervals. Albion was a six-months calf at the time of his purchase, and was bought at sixty guineas ($310), and was of the "alloy" blood; that is, had the strongest outcross in the Colling herd—the strongest of all possible outcrosses, being as it was a cross outside of the breed itself. When put to Halnaby, by Mr. Booth's Lame Bull, this strongest of outcrosses Albion got Young Albion, which proved one of the most splendid of breeders. Then in 1818 Mr. Booth bought at Mr. Robert Colling's sale a yearling bull, Pilot (496), at 270 guineas ($1,400), by Major (398) or Wellington (680), in neither case an extremely in-and-in bred bull for those days, the relationship being aunt or great aunt to nephew, though he had a great deal of Favorite blood, which drew these blood lines much more closely together. This bull was a great sire also, especially doing wonders on the out-blood of the Darlington Market cow in "White Cow," getting Isabella and Own Sister to Isabella and Lady Sarah. Of the earlier crosses used that of Matchem, purchased at Mr. Mason's sale, is esteemed by Mr. Carr the best. The blood of Matchem was used more freely in the herd through his son out of Young Carnation—Young Matchem (4420), his dam being out of Carnation by Pilot. Young Matchem made a deep impression on the herd. These are only specimen and typical examples of the outcrosses used in the Booth herds at Killerby, Studley, and Warlaby. There was a long list of bulls hired and bought from the days of Ben down with out-blood, and they or their get were constantly and freely used. To enumerate but a few of them, there were Mussulman, Leonard, Exquisite, Water King, and Lord Stanley, all of which were brought together to produce those wonderful beasts of our own day, Commander-in-Chief (21451) and Lady Fragrant. Of these Mussulman deserves a passing notice. "It was sufficient for Mr. J. Booth," says Carr, "that he saw in Mussulman not merely the fortuitous possessor of equally valuable properties with those which his own herd could boast, but the inheritor of them, for being descended from the stocks of Messrs. Wright and Charge Mussulman's ancestry had all been well known to Mr. Booth for generations. It has been asserted by overzealous advocates of the system of close interbreeding that the crosses of Mussulman, Lord Lieutenant, Matchem, and others introduced scarcely any fresh blood into the Booth herds; for inasmuch as no alien bulls were used but those whose veins were surcharged with the blood of Favorite, the recourse to them was nothing more than a recurrence to, or renewal of, the old family strain; but this is really only what is true of every well-bred Short-horn of the period, and therefore proves nothing. * * * It will not do, therefore, to claim bulls as of kindred blood on this ground only. Moreover, it must in candor be admitted by the advocates of in-and-in breeding that a careful consideration of the above facts leads to one unavoidable conclusion. Very strong in-and-in breeding is a totally different thing in our case from what it was in the case of the earlier breeders—the Collings and Mr. Thomas Booth—so different that there can be but little analogy between the two cases. They bred in-and-in from animals which had little or no previous affinity. We breed in-and-in from animals full of the same blood to begin with. In our case the *via* *media*, and, therefore, the *via salutis*, would seem to lie in the adoption of two apparently opposite principles—*in-and-in breeding* and *fresh blood*." It is also worth while to note the place which Lord Lieutenant has in the history of the Booth cattle. His significance is manifold. First of all he was an excellent beast. "A short-legged, thick, and lusty dog, but rather lacking in hair," is Mr. Dixon's description of him. Next, in Wm. Raine's rather prejudiced opinion, "Booth never had a good bull till he used Lord Lieutenant," and thus got Leonard. Next he, like all of Mr. Raine's cattle, was a wonderfully well-bred bull, being crowded with the best old blood brought in through cross after cross. Still, again, it is significant that this good bull, excellent breeder, and immortal sire of Leonard was full of the blood of St. John (572), which bull Mr. Bates thought so ill of, though if the descendants of Leonard are any criterion of what St. John's blood was able to do for cattle it is a pity that we have not more of it. Lastly and chiefly, Lord Lieutenant is remarkable as having effected one of the most important outcrosses ever put on the Booth herd. He was brought in to preserve the stamina and give a fresh impulse to the herd, which was needing it badly. Clearly up to this time both the brothers—John and Richard Booth—believed and acted on the faith that at occasional intervals a fresh strain of blood was necessary to the health and profit of the herd. Mr. Richard Booth was not so staunch after Exquisite failed to "nick" to suit him, yet through his exquisite judgment and the sturdiness of his stock, already full of the out-blood of Lord Lieutenant, Mussulman, Water King, Exquisite, and Lord Stanley, he was able to put off the evil day till after his time; but Nemesis was not to follow his course in vain, and she wreaked her revenge when his successor was forced to incorporate the Torr cattle with his herd because of impaired fecundity. It was Richard Booth who first sent White Strawberry to Lord Lieutenant in 1839, though it was John Booth who apparently selected both Lord Lieutenant and Mussulman as the bulls with which to introduce fresh blood into their herds. Whoever made the choice it was made "with infinite judgment," says Mr. Dixon, and the event justifies his opinion; moreover, there was, until a somewhat later date, no difference in opinion or practice between the brothers. It was only as Richard grew into old age that he changed his practice radically. This divergence was no doubt largely the result of natural disposition. Richard Booth is said to have been "a dignified recluse, and thought there was no place like home"; while John was always fond of going about to shows and visiting about among other farmers and breeders. Naturally the one drifted, as did Mr. Bates, to place an over-estimate on his own cattle and an undervaluation on those of others; while the other maintained a more healthful mental atmosphere and juster judgment. It is sufficiently evident, surely, that while the Booths inbred they never ceased to recognize its dangers nor to actively fight them with strong outside blood until after many years, and that the abandonment of the constant recourse to fresh blood led to disaster. Nevertheless a single example, traced for a period of years through a number of generations, may make this somewhat clearer.

We have seen that the direct outcross of the Colling bull Pilot on the "White Cow" with a single cross produced the celebrated Isabella. She was bred to Young Matchem by the Mason outcross Matchem, and produced Isabella Matchem. Isabella Matchem was bred to the bull Leonard by the Raine outcross Lord Lieutenant, and produced Fitz Leonard, who was the sire of the great sire Crown Prince. Isabella Matchem, with her two outcrosses, was also bred three times to Buckingham, son of the Craddock outcross Mussulman, and produced the celebrated bull Vanguard, "a noble bull, as all the Buckingham bulls were"; Insurance, which produced to Leonard, son of the outcross Lord Lieutenant, Leonidas, "a very fine bull, sire of the notable Monk, one of the best of the Warlaby bulls," and Isabella Buckingham. To the outcross Exquisite she also produced Isabella Exquisite. Isabella Buckingham, with her three outcrosses, is said to have been "a superb cow." She produced to the strong outcross Exquisite, Sample (four outcrosses), which, though a plain cow herself, like all of Exquisite's get, was, like most of them, a fine breeder, and produced to Hopewell Isabella Hopewell, a beautiful animal, and to Crown Prince Lady Grace, another of Mr. Booth's best cows. Hopewell was himself by the outbred bull Buckingham, dam by the outbred bull Leonard, grandam by the outbred bull Young Matchem; while Crown Prince was by Fitz Leonard, the breeding of which has already been noticed, and his dam was the cow Charity by the outbred bull Buckingham, grandam by the outbred bull Young Matchem.

In fine we see that the Booths, like Mr. Bates, confined their breeding as far as possible to their own herd in the main, but they took care to infuse an abundance of strong, fresh, unrelated blood into the home-bred sires used by them by means of radical outcrosses. That this was the means which enabled them to breed the fine cattle which they so constantly bred is, in view of the facts, impossible to doubt. Among the more notable of the living breeders of Short-horn cattle Mr. Amos Cruickshank, of Aberdeenshire, holds a prominent place. He shares with the Messrs. Colling, Booth, and Bates the honor of having formed a distinct type within the breed, and of having given to this type his own name, so that the expression "Cruickshank cattle" is quite as familiar today as "Booth bred" or as "Bates strain." He stands as sponsor to a type that has been steadily growing in popularity in Great Britain and America for a number of years past, and as an admirable example of a more recent breeder than those already named, who has fallen under the same temptation to which they were subjected, of making a close sub-breed of his cattle. Some account of his breeding methods has seemed likely to further illustrate this subject.

It is now more than fifty years since Mr. Cruickshank began his career as a breeder. That beginning was of the most modest kind. In 1837 he made a trip to Durham and took back with him to Scotland a single Short-horn heifer. He was then a young man. The son of a farmer in the neighborhood of Inverarie, he had inherited the sturdy Scotch character, and had been brought up in the rather stern school of Scotch agricultural experience. About the time of the purchase of this first heifer he had taken the large farm of Sittyton, a then unknown name, which he has rendered familiar to all breeders of Short-horn cattle. His Scotch temperament caused him to "make haste slowly," and with his one heifer and her produce he was content for some time, but soon began a system of judicious purchases wherever good cattle were to be found, buying the best, both bulls and cows. From the outset he bought those that spoke for themselves. Individual merit was his great object. Consequently an examination of his herd's record, even in the fourth and fifth decades of the century, reveals many prize-winners, both among the animals purchased from time to time and also among the animals of his own breeding. Indeed, from the very outset this herd took its place among the prize-winning herds, and has won innumerable triumphs both in England and Scotland. This speaks clearly enough for the character of stock chosen by Mr. Cruickshank. An inspection of the pedigrees of the animals further shows how good was the judgment displayed in selecting the stock. Many fancies have had their day in the past fifty years. They have come and gone, leaving often scarcely the least memory of their existence. Mr. Cruickshank seems to have pandered to none of them. He chose for the foundations of many of the families with which he has been most successful pedigrees which the votaries of one or another of the then existing fashions would have said were very plain. Breeders were then, as now, stumbling over that difficulty. There were any number of wiseacres about to warn men against this or that pedigree because it was plain or unfashionable; but the so-called plain-bred cattle were certainly good, and the fashionable strains were far from always being so, and Mr. Cruickshank was too good a judge and too clear-headed a business man to be affected by mere fine-spun theories. He had even so early as this gotten a good hold upon the idea that personal merit and descent from animals of the same sort was the only bovine aristocracy which was capable of enduring the wear and tear of time, and making that his test he hewed to the line. There was no iconoclasm or fanaticism in all this. He made no comments or criticism on the follies of the day. While he did not shrink from the most neglected stock if they only showed a substantial pedigree and that substance in the personal qualifications which was a *sine qua non* with him, he yet was always ready to recognize the good in the most fashionable strains when it really existed, and purchased and used some highly fashionable bulls. In this he was in exact line with Mr. Thomas Booth's most notable example.

As year after year passed, and animal after animal was purchased on account of excellence in this or that direction, because of show-yard triumphs, and other like grounds of sound reason, many and various strains very naturally found their way into the herd. It was a kind of natural selection on a high standard which drew from far and wide. Among these purchases we find animals descended from the good old-fashioned sorts of Maynard, Colling, Mason, and Wetherell; newer sorts from the herds of Booth and Bates; and every variety of blood in one bull and another, at the foundation or brought in by top crosses. A notable strain, among others, of Col. Towneley's was the Barmpton Rose (certainly one of the best of the good old families), introduced chiefly in Master Butterfly 2d, a $2,000 bull "of great individual merit," while others came from such herds as those of Messrs. Torr, Stuart, William Smith, Linton, Capt. Barclay, Sir William Sterling Maxwell, and Earl Ducie. Wherever they could be found to come up to the one clearly fixed and high standard they were purchased, if possible, and mere theories counted for nothing.

This process went on for about thirty years. After so long a time the herd had grown large, even very large, and by the constant introduction of new strains, through the purchase of cows and the purchase and hiring of bulls, the animals were as thoroughly miscellaneous in their breeding as it was possible for them to be. For a long period scarcely a year passed without the introduction of some new strain. During all this time the herd had steadily gained in reputation. This was often and plainly shown by the large prices realized at various sales. Nor was the success in the more important direction of securing and maintaining the excellence in form and quality, which Mr. Cruickshank made his principal aim, less notable. None who saw the herd questioned the success of the effort to breed a fine type of easy-feeding, short-legged, deep-fleshed butcher's beasts.

After so long a time, when the excellence and the fame of the herd were placed on so sure a footing, when Mr. Cruickshank was himself well past the meridian of life and might naturally think the time had come to reap as thoroughly as possible the results of his labors and reputation, a change of method was inaugurated. But this change was neither radical nor violent. The constant introduction of all kinds of fresh blood from any and every source was given up. The only rule of practice hitherto discernible was the gathering in of the best animals anywhere to be found. This led to an extreme form of outbreeding, followed not because it was outbreeding, but chiefly because it was the only means by which the Sittyton herd could secure the best that England and Scotland produced. But none the less while these models of excellence were being secured the highest advantages of the outbreeding or natural method were gained. The constant infusion of fresh, vigorous strains from widely separated districts made the herd one of the most vigorous in the land. While other herds were growing smaller every year, were showing broad marks of enfeeblement, and were wasting to a bare skeleton of what they once had been, this one had grown from 1837 to 1870 to one of the most numerous and one of the most vigorous in Great Britain. It was under such circumstances that Mr. Cruickshank began to use almost exclusively home-bred bulls. But he fell into no incestuous breeding. His herd was large, full of many strains, and as fresh in blood as were the cattle which Maynard and Colling and Booth began their careers with. The famous Champion of England (17526), regarded by Mr. Cruickshank not merely as the best breeder he ever bred, but even as the best he ever used, began the new regime. From his time of service dates the beginning of nearly twenty years of effort to breed not only fine animals but also animals of a common type. In his object of fixing a common type upon his stock Mr. Cruickshank has been greatly favored by a long and vigorous life, and he has been wise enough never to sacrifice individual quality to type character. The destruction of many who began well lay in adopting the opposite course. Mr. Cruickshank has studiously avoided the pitfalls of in-and-in and incestuous methods of breeding, and has worked consistently along broad and well-marked lines.

As has already been indirectly pointed out, no argument is needed to establish the certainty of the success of Mr. Cruickshank as a breeder. The records of his herd in the show-yard and his well-established reputation both witness very strongly to this, which those who have seen any large number of his cattle do not need to have proved. But there is one fact in this connection which is worthy of notice, and which certainly tends to enhance the importance of the success and reputation which the Sittyton herd has won, and that is that while the great majority of the herds which have won permanent fame have been located in or near that little corner of England to which the Short-horn belonged in primitive times, this herd has risen, thriven, and grown famous away up in the northern part of Scotland where the granite hills are bare to the bleak winds of the Northern Ocean. There was no prestige of neighborhood or antecedents. What has been won has been won by honest effort. The only materials used have been good cattle, sound principles, and hard work, and with them a worthy fabric has been reared.

And passing this notable example we may read the same lesson in the work that has been done and is being done by many contemporary breeders. To every one who has been alive to the recent tendencies of breeding in England, especially as shown in the show-yard, the growth of a body of very successful exhibitors who used the great rule of merit for merit's sake must have been obvious. Among these the name of Wm. Duthie of Collynie, Aberdeenshire, a neighbor, and in some points a disciple, of Mr. Cruickshank, has been especially notable. He has used many of Mr. Cruickshank's cattle and some of his theories with marked advantage. His fine stock bull Field Marshal, which American buyers several times sought to bring to this country in vain, was not long since hired to the Queen for use in the Royal herd, which well illustrates how the Northern fame and Northern cattle are winning ground. Among other breeders who seem to have much the same views of the true method of breeding may be named such well-known and successful breeders as Messrs. Brierly, Garne, Handley, R. Stratton, and Hutchinson. With such men coming so prominently to the front, both in Scotland and in England, it is perhaps not unreasonable to expect that the next period of breeding will be one characterized by very general miscellaneous breeding. There are very few men in this day of anything even remotely approaching extended experience who would for a moment advocate or indulge in incestuous breeding to any great extent. The most that is now met with is line breeding carried to so close a degree as to be inbreeding, at least to a limited extent.

To sum up, then: the historical testimony drawn from the practice of the most famous breeders is to the effect that incestuous breeding was tried and found after a very short time to be, even in the hands of the most skillful breeders, an utter failure and a ruin to many cattle; that outcrosses are necessary not only in order to maintain the constitutional vigor of the cattle, but also to secure the best general results; that all, or nearly all, breeders have abandoned the close methods of breeding as too dangerous to be risked, even when believed to be, as they still are by some, the surest road to occasional phenomenal results.

The gardener and the scientist find that the most radical outcrosses, even to the extent of hybridism, are the roads to really valuable variation to better types. The history of

Short-horn breeding is certainly a record of the need of frequent and vigorous outcrosses, and is written more in the names of such bulls as Hubback, Belvedere, Lord Lieutenant, and Champion of England than such as Comet and Treble Gloster.

CROSS BREEDING.

Cross breeding is, properly speaking, the mating of animals of distinct breeds. There has been not a little confusion in late years produced by a want of clear distinctions in terms used in breeding. The analogy between the relations of family to family and tribe to tribe and that of breed to breed has naturally led to the use of terms, especially in the absence of others more accurate, properly belonging to the wider sphere in a restricted sense. Thus we hear of cross breeding in the limits of particular breeds, as of a cross of Booth upon Bates. It is so essential to the intelligent discussion of any subject that the terminology shall be exact and generally accepted, that all such looseness of speech must be deplored, even while we find how hard it is to avoid it.

I here use cross breeding in its true and original signification—the mating of animals of distinct breeds. We have two divisions of this subject forced on us by modern conditions which are quite distinct and require to be looked at from totally different points of view. In the first place we have crosses between two distinct breeds where the breeds are both well recognized improved breeds; and secondly, crosses between an improved breed and a native, or unimproved stock. The conditions of the two methods of crossing are quite different. The latter we usually speak of as "grading-up" and the resulting offspring we call "grades." The former is most distinctively termed "crossing" and the resulting products are called "crosses" or "cross-bred cattle."

Cross breeding in its narrower sense of crosses between two distinct breeds of improved stock has lost much of its importance on account of the great value which is now put upon pedigree. Pedigree and the absolute purity of blood, to say nothing of the demand so often made for a single, or at most a few strains of ultra-fashionable blood, have in recent years been so much the dominant features of cattle-breeding as to make it almost impossible for any breeder to go contrary to the popular tendency. The tendency of an earlier day was quite the reverse. There was a general sentiment prior to the time of Bakewell, the Collings, and other contemporary or nearly contemporary improvers, that the cattle and domestic animals as they then existed were of a poor quality and could be and ought to be improved. How to do this was the question, and the general sentiment of the time adopted the idea of crossing breed with breed. At one time it was carried to an immoderate extent, and in the hands of ignorant experimenters all manner of errors were committed, and these mistakes not infrequently led to serious permanent harm.. Other breeders of more wisdom and judgment proceeded with more care and doubtless did not a little to improve the different breeds of stock. The breed lines in many cases were at that time much less closely drawn than at the present day. The types were far less artificially differentiated nearly everywhere. If, however, it is true, as maintained by Darwin, Rütimeyer, and other men of science, that the European breeds of cattle are descended from three aboriginal and quite distinct species, then it is likely that in some cases there were more extreme differences among European cattle in an earlier day than exist now, and it is perhaps to the constant experimentation with cross breeding that we owe the assimilation to a general type which existed in the early part of the eighteenth century and which more readily yielded to variation than could have been expected from the original type. However this may be, up to the time of Bakewell improvement was chiefly sought through crosses, and this method had the approval of all classes; of scientists and theoretical writers as well as experimenters and practical farmers.

A wise man and judicious breeder who had made a thoughtful study and a careful analysis of the character of the stock from which he was breeding, and who clearly saw that a defect in one breed was to be amended by seeking another breed with a corresponding excellence in that point, and who blended and waited patiently for the result, not expecting too much from the first generation, often secured very good results. But the work thus accomplished was occasional and spasmodic, and the results as recorded and finally summed up in history are without evidence of any material progress. The most that can be claimed for the epoch is that it was a period of preparation during which the theatre was being made ready and the instruments prepared for the activities of the succeeding age.

The progress made by individual breeders must have oftentimes seemed of a high degree, otherwise it is impossible to see why this method was so long adhered to to the exclusion of every other. It has been well settled that such crosses are very fruitful in vigor and vitality. It was perhaps this which tempted the unsatisfied experimenters on, and still on, even when the ultimate results were not what was looked for.

It thus soon became necessary to come to some sort of definite conception as to a permanent method. Was there to be a constant and continuous interfusion of the blood of two or more breeds, or were the results of the first series of crosses to be made the basis of a new breed, or was the cross to be introduced merely as an occasional remedy for some particular fault which, once done, the regular line of the breed upon which the cross was made would be returned to?

The first of these methods lacks any motive for its adoption, and is too little susceptible of systematization to seriously attract any practical breeder who aims to attain a real improvement. The second was naturally a favorite with many of the more ambitious experimenters, but the verdict of posterity seems to be that in most animals the effort to keep up a breed formed by intercrossing any two given breeds, where no other method was used in conjunction with it, has not been especially successful save in a very few cases, which are notable rather as exceptions than as antagonistic facts. It is to be kept in mind that this is not meant to cover such cases as those in which a special quality has been obtained by means of a cross and perpetuated by resort to the Bakewell methods. The line of distinction lies in the method of selection chiefly. In one case the basis of the selection consists of all animals which are cross bred in a particular manner; in the other only such of the special cross-bred type as are possessed of the certain special features for which the cross was made. In the one case the descendants all are within the class; in the other each successive generation must be carefully culled of all failing to conform to the standard. If the qualities prove non-transmissible and die out in the one case the variety lives on as an empty name; in the other it ceases for the lack of a *raison d'etre.* It is very doubtful if there is any recognized distinct breed formed of the union of two other original breeds which can be traced to a simple mixing of the breed and subsequent breeding from all sprung from the cross.

By far the most usual course pursued in making crosses is the third method. It was eminently natural for a breeder whose stock showed a particular defect to seek a male of another breed which did not have a like fault and make a cross upon his stock with him in the hope of curing the deficiency. The cross once made, the ordinary course of breeding within the old breed would be returned to.

A somewhat remarkable example—though a legitimate offspring of the time and place, and not a mere experiment—of the first method took place in Kentucky in early times. A few head of cattle—some Short-horns and some Longhorns—were imported to Maryland and

Virginia, and thence a few head passed, through the instrumentality of the Messrs. Patton, to Kentucky. This was between 1783 and 1800, and none of the stock was very highly improved, except that it is just possible that the Longhorns may have felt the impetus of Bakewell's work. These cattle were interbred without regard to the distinctions of breed, and as they were few and the early cows neither very prolific nor very fortunate in producing females, a hodge-podge of Short-horn and Longhorn was made, all somewhat diluted by native blood. No chance was lost to make a cross with bulls of either of the original breeds, and at a later time Hereford blood was probably added to the mixture. The cattle known as "Patton stock" were very decidedly superior to the common native stock, and it was much esteemed and sought after; but after 1817, when the number of pure-bred cattle in the State began to be considerable, they rapidly sank out of sight as they could not bear the competition with the pure-bred stock.

The famous Kentucky importation of 1817 also consisted of Longhorns and Short-horns, which in some cases were interbred; but no new Longhorn blood being brought to America the produce all came to Short-horn bulls, and the Longhorn blood sank out of sight, and the status of the cattle was changed to the third case, where a cross is made and then a return is had to a single breed exclusively. In the same year (1817) Hon. Henry Clay imported some Hereford cattle to Kentucky, and they, too, after being crossed impartially with Short-horns and Longhorns and mixed Longhorn-Short-horn bulls, passed out of sight, being lost in the ever-increasing tide of Short-horn blood.

Crosses have been very extensively used by sheep-breeders to improve and modify their flocks; so much so that most of the cultivated breeds have at one time or another suffered an infusion of alien blood

For instance, the Hampshire sheep were originally horned, large, and coarse. In order to improve them a movement began, soon after the great improving impulse of the last century had reached a good development and shown what it was possible to do in bettering the character of the British flocks, by using South-down rams in the flocks. The cross proved a happy one and the Hampshire breed was certainly improved by it. They are now finer in the bone, wider in the back, rounder in the barrel, and of better quality; and, moreover, have lost their horns, being in this particular assimilated to the Southdown type.

Again, in Wiltshire we have a somewhat similar method. In that country "where the same old horned stock originally prevailed the improved Southdown gradually took the place of the old breed, which soon disappeared. The imported Southdown ewes were after a time crossed with improved Hampshire rams that already had a large proportion of Southdown blood, for the purpose of giving an increase in size,"* and crossing of a more or less radical nature has been used in developing very nearly all the breeds of English sheep. The Cheviots, for instance, have been used on a number of mountain varieties, and it is said that the Cheviots have themselves been repeatedly crossed with other breeds for their own advantage. Among those thus used the Leicesters and the Cotswolds may be mentioned.

The distinct character of the breeds of sheep naturally invited crossing. The great differences in quantity and quality of wool and in capacity to fatten and in the quality of the meat among the better breeds, suggested that a wise intermingling of the blood of several varieties might lead to a combination that would be profitable to the general farmer. The high excellence of some of the breeds of middle-wool sheep doubtless was partly a resultant of this circumstance. Even more natural was it that some of the hardy but diminutive and otherwise inferior mountain varieties should be improved so far as they

* Miles on "Stock-Breeding," cited from "Journal of the Royal Agricultural Society."

would bear it by crosses with the more valuable sorts. As the conditions of life were improving for all domestic animals about this time such improvement was rarely at the cost of destroying the capacity of the flocks to thrive in their environment. Such crosses were used on Welsh and Scotch breeds in the main with great advantage. There was some trouble at first in the cross of the Cheviot with the Black-faced Heath breed in Scotland, so much so that Youatt says: "The black-faced sheep seemed obstinately to resist the influence of foreign crosses. The Leicester and even the Cheviot blood added little to the value of either the fleece or the carcass, while they materially lessened the hardihood of the sheep." There seems to have been a general misunderstanding of the manner of making the crosses at first, and it was noted at the time that the winters were exceptionally severe at the period during which the crosses were being made. It appears that at first those showing the utmost Cheviot character were always the ones reserved for breeding, "while the figure, wool, and other qualities of the Cheviot rams were most conspicuous in the smallest and feeblest of the progeny" in the first cross; "while the properties of the mountain breed were more fully exhibited in the strongest and most robust of the lambs. This misled many of the storemasters. They did not consider that there was as much Cheviot blood in the coarsest (as they were pleased to call them) as in the finest, though not so clearly exhibited in its external qualities. This induced them to throw aside the best of the lambs and select those to breed from which had apparently most of the Cheviot figure." The true method for the breeders to have pursued was to select the most vigorous of the ewe lambs and to continue the use of pure Cheviot rams till the wool and flesh were improved without any loss of physical vigor. Although thus somewhat discouraged the interfusion of the Cheviot blood was persisted in till a large proportion of the flocks of the old black-faced sheep had been supplanted by cross-bred or purely-bred Cheviot stock.

Many varieties of swine have arisen from crosses of breed with breed, and the same system has at one time or another been tried more or less widely on almost all farm stock. Sometimes where the animals produced are hybrids and infertile, crosses are resorted to on account of the vigor of the produce. The mule—resulting from a cross between the jack and mare—is the best known of these cases. A cross between any of the ordinary breeds of the domestic duck with a Muscovy drake has been frequently used to secure a large and very easily fattened hybrid fowl for table use.

These crosses are necessarily outside of our purview.

An interesting chapter of Short-horn history resulted from a cross made in early days by two gentlemen, one of whom was the celebrated improver Mr. Charles Colling. About the year 1791 Col. O'Calahan, a neighbor of Mr. Colling's, bred a red polled Galloway heifer to Mr. Colling's bull Bolingbroke (86), and she produced a bull calf known as "Son of Bolingbroke." This bull was bred to Johanna by Lame Bull (358), and produced a bull calf known as Grandson of Bolingbroke. Both of these bulls were recorded in the English Short-horn Herd Book, with the numbers (469) and (280). The last named bull was put to Phœnix, the dam of Favorite (252), and got the heifer calf Lady, which produced a number of calves to Colling's most esteemed sires, such as Favorite (252), Cupid (177), and Comet (155). This family, on account of the Galloway blood, came to be known as the "alloy," and the cattle were certainly very good ones, and as the lines of purity of blood were not very strictly drawn at that time no special attention was paid to the cross. At the great closing-out sale in 1810 some nineteen head of cattle with the Galloway cross in them were sold at an average price of about one hundred and thirty-eight guineas, or about seven hundred dollars, one of them reaching four hundred guineas, a little more than two thousand dollars. Some time after the sale discussion arose on the subject, some claiming that the cross was made for the distinct purpose of effecting an improvement, and that a real improvement was caused by it. The celebrated pamphlet of the Rev. Henry Berry took this ground. Most Short-horn breeders, however, took the position that it had been done without any serious purpose, that the stock proving good Mr. Colling had retained it and used his Short-horn bulls on it with no thought of repeating the experiment, and that so small was the infusion of alien blood, and so thoroughly had it been crossed out, that it was a matter of little moment one way or another. The effort to discredit the blood was only partially successful, and we find it in the herds of such breeders as Sir H. Vane Tempest and Mr. Bates. Mr. Bates came out at length against it, though he urgently advised the agents of the Ohio Importing Company, in 1834, to purchase of him a bull which had the alloy cross. It is so far behind us that the "alloy" is now only an interesting episode in Short-horn history.

The interest in crosses has been somewhat reawakened by the success in recent years of cross-bred animals in the fat-stock shows at Chicago and Kansas City. These crosses have mainly resulted, not from any intentional experimentation with cross breeding, but rather from high grades of one breed being bred as grades to bulls of other breeds. There may be some exceptions to this, but in the main this is true, and they are classed in the shows with grades. Among these animals there have been quite a variety of breeds represented, and many combinations of blood have been presented. The principal breeds have been the three great beef breeds—the Short-horn, the Hereford, and the polled Angus. We find, also, the Galloway, the West Highland, and the Devon breed in a few cases. Among these there have been several animals of very high excellence which were crosses of Short-horn and Hereford, sometimes with some native blood also, and quite a large number of a cross between the Angus and the Short-horn. The steer Plush was a successful mixture of Devon with Hereford blood; while the phenomenal steer Nigger showed how excellently, at least in his case, a mixture of Hereford and Angus blood had resulted.

Whether these cases of extraordinary results produced by crossing different breeds will ever take form in any practical experiments to determine the value of such crosses for producing cattle for the beef market may well be doubted. The method of grading as a subordinate department of cross breeding has been found to yield such excellent results that it is likely long to remain the popular process of bettering the character of market cattle. It is still more unlikely that any combination of existing breeds will be made for the purpose of producing a new distinct breed. The various breeds have attained so high a state of excellence in differentiation and adaptation to the ends for which they are in demand, while the Shorthorn still maintains in such a high degree its excellence as a general-purpose beast for the farmer, that men are not likely to be distracted from slow but sure improvement of these highly improved breeds in a vain, or at best a long, slow, and unpromising attempt to reach an end already sufficiently attained.

The interest, then, for the cattle-breeder in cross breeding is largely historical and monitory. In it he sees a system—one highly esteemed and fully tried; one capable in wise hands of producing some good, but in the main tending rather to no permanent good result.

GRADE BREEDING.

We have seen already that cross breeding was properly divisible into two classes—the interbreeding of two distinct breeds or varieties where both were improved breeds, and the interbreeding of one such breed with an unimproved or native stock. We have now to discuss the latter method.

This breeding of one animal of an improved breed with another of an unimproved or native stock is usually spoken of as grading or grading up. By grading is meant a leveling, step by step—by gradations, to use a word of exactly similar derivation. This grading is just the same process as the word signifies when we apply it to mechanical work, as grading a street. It is, however, here used in the sense of leveling up. Hence the frequent use of the additional preposition "up." The aim is not merely to level, as is most commonly done in mechanical work by getting a mean between the highest and lowest points—though this is not infrequently all that is really attained—but the aim is to raise the average to the maximum and to make the grade level with the highest point. In short, to make a "fill" rather than a "grade," in engineering parlance. But of course no analogy ever quite exactly fits, and so if we run on after our analogy here we will only obscure the idea which we wish to elucidate. The process itself is simple enough, and the object and its *raison d'etre* equally obvious.

The improved breeds are all of much higher excellence in their special spheres than are the best of native stocks in an unimproved condition. They are thoroughly adapted to the demands of the varied life of man, and the stock raisers who are the purveyors to those demands whenever they are alive to their own best interests are eager to avail themselves of the excellences which these breeds possess. There are not, however, nearly enough animals of these improved breeds to supply the demand for man's use. If the pure-bred Herefords, Short-horns and Angus should be devoted to supplying the beef trade they would in a short time all be slaughtered and cease to exist. They are only as yet numerous enough to supply the demand for cattle for fancy breeding as opposed to market breeding; that is to say, for breeding purposes as opposed to consumption. But there must be some practical basis of utility outside and beyond this mere breeding to give it an object and to give the stock a market value. For value is made up of two elements, the first of which is utility, and the second cost, or the labor necessary to produce the article. What, then, is this outside utility?

It is based, first, on the need of those who supply the market to have the best possible products with which to meet its demand. Competition here, as everywhere else, drives the weaker to the wall, while that best fitted to supply the need of man survives. There is a limit put to the price which can be obtained for such market products, however, by man's wealth and ability to pay. While the best will always command the highest price in the market, it will not be an extravagant price under ordinary circumstances. The products with which the market is supplied, as soon as absolute necessaries are passed, are regulated by the price which can be obtained for them. That is to say, the market product is first demanded for its utility. Whether that demand can be supplied depends, secondly, on whether it can be produced at a cost less than the price at which there is a demand for it. It is perfectly obvious that if I cannot produce Durham beef at less than $200 per head for two-year-old beasts, and they only bring $100 for consumption, and the demand for then is at that sum and no more, the market will be unsupplied. Men will be forced to take the best they can get at that price, or a little lower if they can get it.

But price is regulated by utility and cost, being merely value in terms of money. Hence the utility of an animal of a beef breed we may fairly say is its capacity to make good beef. It would be gauged by the demand for beef thus far. But cost means the labor necessary to produce a given article: that is, to raise a cow or steer, and we know that a cow or steer can be raised and sold at a profit at the market rate. What, then, is the reason that a Durham steer cannot be disposed of at the market shambles at the market price? Simply this: "Labor necessary to produce a given article" includes the whole labor. Thus as to gold it includes the labor of discovery as well as that of mining and working, etc.; so that in one sense the scarcity of a product is an element in the cost. Hence the labor in producing a Durham steer includes all the labor of the wise improvers who put labor of the most highly-skilled sort into the work of improving the breed. Every bit of all the labor put forth in thus developing his ancestry counts in his price. These steers are scarce then. There are few that have so much labor put on them; if it were not so the labor so expended would have lacked a proper return to justify its expenditure. The production is always limited, too—limited by the number of animals possessing this form of value, and limited by the ability of those persons engaged in multiplying this form of product to maintain the excellence once given it; for it is obvious that if a product is valued for the labor expended on it by nine workmen, and when passed into the hands of a tenth, he, by his want of skill, not only does not improve the article but spoils that which was done by his predecessors, he has decreased rather than increased the value of the article. His labor has, as the mathematicians say, a negative value; he has added work but not productive labor. So an unskillful breeder may wreck the work of many generations of skillful breeders, and at a stroke reduce cattle of the highest quality, in their descendants, to the rank of mere beef cattle. This is no more labor than the muscular exertion required to knock the head of a statue by Praxitiles from the shapely shoulders would be labor. It requires real, productive labor to maintain the excellence produced originally with so much difficulty in our improved breed.

Not only so but the females are the sole source of pure descent when mated with pure males—their production is limited to not more than one animal per annum, and half of these on the average will be bulls. The bulls being thus one-half and their productive capacity being, let us say, fifty fold that of the cows, their demand for the purposes of breeding thoroughbred cattle is approximately as one to fifty. That is, only one bull is required for every fifty cows. From such a conclusion in the abstract we would think that a bull would be worth one-fiftieth as much as a cow. But we bethink ourself of the demand for market beef and we conclude with this additional idea in our minds that every bull if steered would be worth as much as a first-class steer at market rates. So we would expect the value of the cows to be regulated by the demand for thoroughbred breeding purposes, and that of the bulls to be about one-fiftieth of that, or the market price of steers, whichever was highest.*

But we discovered in our study of the laws of animal prepotency that a breed deeply bred in a fixed type was prepotent over a heterogeneous or native type. And so the breeder of mere market cattle, being anxious to attain the highest market price for his stock, is driven by keen competition to seek to improve his stock. The demand he has to meet does not justify him if he is a breeder of market cattle in buying at an outlay of thousands of dollars thoroughbred stock, however desirable. But as a thoroughbred bull begets animals greatly resembling himself he is justified in buying such a bull and using him on his common stock. Here,

*There is really another element which sometimes occurs in such a case to alter the value, but it is not important in the present discussion.

then, is the great source of demand which keeps the demand for thoroughbred beef-bulls closely equal and sometimes above that of the females.

The philosophy of grading rests on the most solid basis of theory and experiment. The scientifically deduced conclusions from the laws of heredity, especially of prepotency, give the highest probability that the offspring of a high-bred bull and a native cow will resemble the bull, and that if this produce is bred back to a high-bred bull and the process continued for a few generations the animals resulting from this course of breeding will be rapidly assimilated to the highly-bred type. To these conclusions practical experiment lends the fullest confirmation. I have bred many grades, many more have been bred under my immediate observation, and I can witness, more especially in the case of Short-horn grades, to the rapidity with which the process of assimilation goes on. As it has been said that bulls vary greatly in prepotency, so also in individual excellence, we would naturally expect great variation in the excellence attained by grading with different bulls. I have already alluded to a phenomenal case of a first cross by the bull Renick on a brindled milch cow; such cases are naturally rare. The second and third crosses on good native cows by really good Short-horn bulls almost always yield animals which even an expert judge could scarcely tell from thoroughbred animals.

Why, then, is the grade not equal to the thoroughbred? For market purposes a high grade, generally speaking, probably is. The taint is in the blood, not in the flesh or form. Interbreed grade with grade and deterioration rapidly follows. The great principle in breeding high-class grades for beef or milk, then, is always to use thoroughbred sires, and never by any means to use a grade bull to breed from.

Why this is so is obvious enough. We have seen that every animal is the joint product of his ancestors, and also that the tendency of all qualities obtained by artificial cultivation is to decline when neglected; all improved breeds constantly inclining to the original type. Consequently, when a grade bull is used on grade cows the tendency is to lose by frequent dilution the moiety of improved blood, and also the further tendency to a general decline to the native type is present in connection with the former, and acts in conjunction with it and gives it a cumulative force. He who tries a cross of high-bred stock on his native cattle is nearly always delighted with the result; so delighted oftentimes that, choosing the most promising of his half-bred bull calves, he uses him as a sire. Disappointment nearly always ensues, and a misconception of the real value of grading up follows. Others use a bull of improved stock for several generations, and then select a bull of their high grades to breed from. In this way they put off the day of reckoning, for a bull of three pure crosses is often a good breeder; but his get in native cows will have only half as much improved blood as he has, and will show it, in most cases, in the herd. The use of grade bulls is, then, a dangerous and condemnable practice, and one to be carefully shunned. The grade cows are to be kept and constantly crossed and re-crossed, generation by generation, with improved bulls. The practice, therefore, which is followed in some of the agricultural shows, of offering prizes for grade bulls for breeding purposes, and for grade herds and for grade bulls and their get, are of injury rather than advantage to the agricultural interests of the country. The encouragement of raising grade steers and cows is to be highly commended; not so the bulls. Every farmer, on the contrary, should be encouraged to steer every bull as soon as calved, and to maintain and increase every bit of excellence gained by systematic and uninterrupted use of a high-bred bull.

And though we saw in the foregoing chapter that cross-bred animals of different high-bred breeds often possessed great merit, as in the case of the great prize-winning steer at the

Chicago Fat-Stock Show, Regulus, which was out of a grade Short-horn and by a Hereford bull, yet on the whole it is perhaps wisest for the breeder of grades to use only one breed in his work of improving. For, as we have seen already, much care and judgment and knowledge of the different breeds thus crossed is necessary to insure success, and this is rarely possessed by the breeder of grade cattle—indeed, all too rarely by anyone. Thus Sir John Sinclair says in regard to the general subject of crossing two distinct breeds (and what he says is precisely applicable here): "As to any attempt at improvement by crossing two distinct breeds or races, one of which possesses the properties which it is wished to obtain, or is free from the defects which it is desirable to remove, it requires a degree of judgment and perseverance to render such a plan successful as is very rarely to be met with." In the native or unimproved stock the nature is plastic to a much higher degree than in these fixed types of improved stocks, and by the interfusion of first one stock and then another with the native stock the fixity of type is gradually given without losing the evil qualities accompanying the unimproved stock. In some places we find mixtures of Jersey and Hereford, Holstein and Short-horn, and all manner of blood, till it is well-nigh hopeless to try to breed them to a good type.

But by choosing a series of Short-horn sires a herd of grades may readily be built up in a few years scarcely inferior for beef and milk and butter to that grand old breed; so by the use of a series of Jersey bulls native stock may be made famous butter-makers; and so on. What the grade-breeder needs, then, is to use improved bulls, and from only one breed.

The question naturally forces itself on us here: How long is this to be continued? Is there no period at which an animal ceases to be a grade and becomes a pure-bred beast? Truly the mysteries of breeding are great, but the mysteries concerning the words "pure-bred," "thoroughbred," etc., are past finding out.

The product of the first cross will contain one-half native blood; of the second cross, one-quarter; of the third, one-eighth; of the fourth, one-sixteenth; of the fifth, one-thirty-second. By the fifth cross, as will be readily seen, the native blood will be reduced to a very small percentage, and as the pure blood dominates in giving form and character it must assuredly be of very little weight in determining character. In consequence some foreign societies admit animals to record in their publications which show five crosses of recorded sires. Others place what is meant to be a requirement of absolute purity as the requisite of record. Thus unbroken descent from an oriental source was long demanded in the English thoroughbred, and importation from England with an English Herd Book record is still demanded of American Short-horn cattle. Hence the anomaly that one may take a cow in England and put five crosses of recorded bulls on her and her produce and gain admission for the produce in both English and American Herd Books, while a score of crosses of unimpeachable sires will never elevate an original American cow's descendants to the dignity of a herd book entry.

In general it is perhaps safe to say that five crosses of highly-bred bulls give the animal the improved character. I am forced to this conclusion by what I believe to be sufficient evidence. Five crosses of mean bulls—weak, impotent—will do little or no good. I am dealing with normal cases. As a breeder I confess to a love of long, far-drawn pedigrees. I love the old-fashioned sorts which have been long well bred and are deeply dyed in the dear traditions of Short-horn excellence; I love such old stocks as the Princess, losing itself as it does in the far-off dawn of Short-horn history; as the Knightley Cold Creams, as the Booth Bracelets, as the Towneley Butterflys, as the Mason Miss Wileys, and so on; but loving them, seeing in them the highest confirmation of the laws of heredity, I am not blind or prejudiced enough not to be able to see that the bulls of their blood are constantly ennobling less ancient lines by infusions of their blood. Cows of five good crosses will win in the show-ring as individuals, and as dams of two or more offspring; while the best bulls of the same number of crosses will vanquish the most excellently bred, both as individuals and as sires. What more is to be asked? Yet we may not run counter to the standards, and where a thousand crosses on an American foundation are no better than one, we must perforce still count them all as grades. Not less profitable are they for the beef market because they are called grades, nor for the making of butter and cheese. And these purposes of utility in practical affairs are the end and object of the grade's existence. For this end the breeder and raiser of the grades must shape their course, and for it the people at large will encourage them. On the other hand, the breeder of improved stock would encourage them for the demand thus secured for males, and the greater and firmer this demand the more profitable will the breeding of high-bred cattle be.

PEDIGREE.

The instant that an animal distinguishes itself for peculiar excellence of any kind its offspring are regarded as of a specially desirable character. This is simply a recognition of the law that like produces like. The fixedness of this law in the mind of men is always being thus illustrated. This is the basis of pedigree. Because men know that like produces like they expect good produce from good animals, and, in view of this, note the ancestry of every animal sprung of valuable parents. The next step is to carry this on to the third generation where a worthy son has succeeded a noble sire, and so on generation after generation. Pedigree is therefore a record of the ancestry of an animal; a table of descent. Simply this. There is no magic spell in a pedigree, no mysterious influence passing out of it and influencing the animal whose genealogy it contains. It may be a record of good ancestry, it may be—unhappily too often is—a list of bad progenitors.

Naturally in an early day it was not customary to preserve any account of the ancestry of an animal unless it was very distinguished.

Men did not care for a record made up of names unhonored and unworthy, or at best in the broad belt of mediocrity. It was only the offspring of the phenomenally good animals whose record of descent was valued. So not unnaturally a vulgar idea sprang up that to have a pedigree was a mark of distinction; for if the animal was not royally descended no such record would have been preserved at all, but the ancestors would have been permitted to sink into deserved oblivion. From this attitude the transition was easy to a general idea that there was some necessary excellence attached to the pedigree, and thence, to an open valuing of an animal for the pedigree, was a facile progression. The want of logic in such steps is only equaled by the lightness with which they have again and again been taken. We have all known men who endeavor to piece out the small stature accorded to them by Nature with the by-gone greatness of a father or a grandfather. We have all seen men deceived by the pretenses of such men, and toadying to them for this reason, while the soberer heads and clearer judgments of most men have bethought them of the frog that tried to puff himself out to the bulk of the bull. Nor is the case less amusing—though often seen—of a miserable brute being lauded to the skies for no other reason than that some remote ancestor possessed fame and merit, and that this miserable descendant is called by his name.

Pedigree, then, is a mere record of ancestry. In the far past of every improved breed we find a starting point; a name which the merit of him that bore it made descent enough. None knew whence he came, or cared not to record it. Thus we find such a case in the Short-horn line in the Studley Bull. He is only a name, without sire or dam that is known to history. He stands on his own merit, a far-off head-spring of a great and ever-swelling river. Most of his descendants, which were doubtless many, were lost to sight in the world of mediocrity. But a little thin line preserved, perpetuated and glorified this old bull's excellence, and in Hubback won for it fame, and through Favorite and many others his blood has passed into a great part of the improved stock. There were many of his descendants of a pedigree very similar to the line which held the mission of giving fame to it, but the descent was nothing without the qualities of the old sire. The descent only of those which honored it was consequently preserved.

We see, then, that pedigree rests on the idea that "like produces like." Its value, therefore, is consequent upon the truth of the laws of heredity. It is because men expect a good beast from a good beast that they desire to know the sire and dam of every animal they are to breed from. It is because animals through sire and dam inherit the natures and characters of their grandparents that men wish to know of them; it is because they now and again revert to the character of a more remote ancestor that they desire to trace back several generations; it is, further, because they have learned that the longer time and the greater number of generations a family or breed has maintained a certain grade of merit the more surely will each succeeding generation reproduce it, that they seek a pedigree of as great length and far ramifications as possible. All these conclusions are natural and logical deductions from the laws of inheritance.

Is, then, a pedigree a guaranty of excellence? The veriest child knows better. The inference justified by the laws of Nature is no more and no less than the simple proposition that as are the progenitors so will the offspring be. If the ancestors are not good neither will the descendants be. A pedigree made up of fine animals, and only when so composed, may be regarded as a guaranty of individual excellence in the animal to which it belongs.

In the beginning, no doubt, only the descent of animals sprung from superior ancestry was preserved. But even in the case of these the descendants have not always maintained their ancestors excellence. Some have been neglected, and declined from insufficient food or want of other things necessary to vigorous physical existence; some have deteriorated from close interbreeding, while others have suffered from injudicious crosses with inferior stocks. To look at a pedigree, then, only so far as the first half-dozen crosses are concerned, when there are a dozen represented in it, is by no means to know anything of the character of the animal to which it belongs. The early crosses may stand out as the best in all the breed; not a line may run outside of the very choicest strains or be represented by any but a famous name; and yet if the last six crosses are represented by mere names, while the cattle that bore them were poor, underfed, consumptive wrecks, or the victims of other kinds of misfortune or mismanagement, no man could expect, with any justness, good results from such a pedigree. We can only expect good animals from others that are good; and if the two animals in the first generation and the four in the second are bad it is only in rare cases of peculiar change of condition for the better that the excellence of great-grandsires exerts a controlling influence for good in a great-grandson.

If every ancestor in a pedigree, on the other hand, stands for merit of a high class, and these many strains of meritorious blood are all brought together in one animal, then, indeed, is a man justified in expecting a corresponding excellence in the produce of such an animal as the one to which this pedigree belongs. Then the pedigree may fairly be said to be a guaranty of excellence.

To generalize broadly, then, a pedigree is a mere record of an animal's ancestors; the fundamental idea of pedigree is that like produces like, and the value of the pedigree grows out of the fact that we expect an animal to breed according as it is bred, *i. e.*, that its offspring will resemble itself, and as it is a combined likeness of its sire and dam, that its offspring will, in so far, resemble that sire and dam, and so on, hence as are the animals in the pedigree so will the descendants be—good if they are good, bad if they are bad. Therefore it becomes the veriest folly to breed from an inferior animal whose sire and dam were also inferior. Such an animal cannot be expected to breed well. Hence fashions in pedigree often lead to great harm. For if we become so wedded to certain blood lines as to breed to no animal not of those lines the time is almost sure to come when bad animals are used for the sake of their pedigree alone. Oftentimes animals of the temporarily popular strains are so few and so high-priced on that account that men will use them on most excellent stock for the sake of fancy and high prices. Once started the canker eats deeper and deeper. Since defects and diseases are prepotent, as we have seen that they are, a defective bull will sometimes taint a whole herd, and through his get many herds. And so the work goes on till the record contained in the pedigree is a long, sad tale of loss, decline, and decay. This is only too common an occurrence, and few breeders of experience are unfamiliar with the course of decadence under such circumstances.

A pedigree is the simple record of a family's life. The only thing which makes pedigrees difficult to understand by those who have given them little or no study is, first, the abbreviated form in which they are commonly written; and second, the rapid widening out as we ascend to remote ancestors, and the consequent complexity and multiplicity of detail. It is comparatively easy, think most men, to trace a man's genealogy. It comes down the male line and the family name forms an easily-followed clue. The long generations, too, take us back so fast that we can go as far as most men care to go before there is much variety. I say, most men think it is easy so to trace a man's pedigree; but as a matter of fact men do with human pedigrees just as they are apt to do with those of animals—attend to one line to the exclusion of every other—only here it is the male, while in cattle, horses, and the other domestic animals it is the female. Let us see how different the result is. I will take as a specimen the pedigree of Baron Butterfly, my old stock bull, which has already been given in its true or extended form. First we have the form, as used in the records of the breed, which gives the line of descent so abbreviated as to show only the feminine line, thus:

BARON BUTTERFLY 49871,

Red and white, calved May 31, 1882, got by 2d Duke of Grasmere 13961, dam Butterfly by Airdrie Renick 7468—White Wreath by St. Valentine 4348½—Bridal Wreath by Imperial Duke (18083)—imp. Miss Butterfly by Master Butterfly (13311)—Rosa by Baron of Ravensworth (7811)—Briseis by Raree Show (4874)—Bessy by Thick Hock (6601)—Barmpton Rose by Expectation (1988)—by Belzoni (1709)—by Comus (1861)—by Denton (198).

We see that this is a Butterfly taking the name of the imported cow, as is very commonly done in this country, or a Barmpton Rose as this family is called in England. Now turning to the male line see what a very different story we read in the record:

BARON BUTTERFLY 49871,

Red and white, calved May 31, 1882, out of Butterfly—by 2d Duke of Grasmere 13961, out of Grace—by Muscatoon 7057, out of Mazurka 2d—by Royal Oxford (18774), out of Lady of Oxford—by 2d Grand Duke (12961), out of Duchess 64th—by 4th Duke of York (10167), out of Duchess 51st—by 2d Duke of Oxford (9046), out of Oxford 2d—by Duke of Northumberland (1940), out of Duchess 34th—by Belvedere (1706), out of Angelina 2d—by Waterloo (2816), out of Angelina—by Young Wynyard (2859), out of Princess—by Wellington (680), out Wildair—by Comet (155), out of Young Phœnix—by Favorite (252),

out of Phœnix—by Bolingbroke (86), out of Young Strawberry—by Foljambe (263), out of Haughton—by Mr. Richard Barker's Bull (52), out of (by a son of Lakeland's Bull)—by Hill's Red Bull, out of ——.

Could the same thing viewed from different points of view be more opposite? And yet these are equally the pedigree of the bull Baron Butterfly in an abbreviated form, and either form would afford the data for an expanded or full pedigree. Turn to this expanded form as given in diagram on pages 138 and 139, and it will make a still different impression on the uninitiated observer. The brief record thus given, which want of space made unavoidable, might lead such an one to think that this bull, instead of being a Barmpton Rose or Butterfly, was more properly to be reckoned as of the Rose of Sharon family. His sire, 2d Duke of Grasmere 13961; his grandsire, Airdrie Renick 7468; his great-grandsire Airdrie 2478, and his great-great-grandsire, Airdrie 2478, were all of the Rose of Sharon family, and having thus an ancestor in each of the four most recent generations of that family, it would seem that this blood must preponderate. It is true that the line which traced this Rose of Sharon descent would be quite a zig-zag across the pedigree, but it would not be any less the animal's true descent. The fallacy of the conclusion does not lie in the necessity of a zig-zag line to trace out the Rose of Sharon ancestors, but in the fact that these bulls are only Roses of Sharon because they trace in the female line to that imported cow. An exact analysis of the pedigree reveals the fact that in seven generations there are one hundred and twenty-eight parts of blood represented, and that of these this so-called Barmpton Rose has only four parts of that family's blood, and the apparently large infusion of Rose of Sharon (or Bates Red Rose) dwindles to only five; while there are twenty-five parts of Oxford and thirty-eight of Duchess blood. There are in all seventy parts of Bates blood, completely swamping the Towneley modest but excellent foundation blood; which is, indeed, exceeded in the total sum by strains from Mr. Whitaker's herd and by the Princess tribe's contribution, and equaled by that from Mr. Mason's herd. The pedigree is more Duchess than anything else, but is one of those superb compounds of many most admirable strains, none of which were superior to that splendid family whose name this grand bull was proud to wear and honored in the wearing.

We thus conclude that the female side is the important one for the Short-horn record—and the same is true of other breeds of cattle—and hence that the first cow with a name is chosen to designate the tribe—in this case Barmpton Rose—or the imported cow quite as often in this country; hence this family is sometimes called the Butterfly family, from imp. Miss

Butterfly by Master Butterfly. It might have been quite as natural to follow the male line and say the family was of "Dicky Barker's Blacknose" tribe, or of the Oxford tribe from Royal Oxford (18774); and it is worthy of note that the early breeders certainly paid more attention to the bulls as the chief element in the pedigree than to the cows. The present popular form of pedigree was originally drawn out as representing simply a list of bulls used in making successive crosses. The cows were quite neglected. Thus in the earliest time the pedigree of Baron Butterfly would have simply been given as by 2d Duke of Grasmere by Airdrie Renick, by St. Valentine, by Imperial Duke, and so on. And the pedigree of each of these bulls would be given the same way. Hence in many pedigrees the early cows are merely represented by dashes; even now in England it is far from uncommon to give the names of the top cows for a few generations and to represent the more remote ancestresses, though their names are perfectly well known, by dashes. The sire was the important factor; to him alone was the number given which made accuracy of reference certain. The sires were regarded as the fountains of all the blood, and it was of no consequence in most cases what the foundation cow might be. The names of the dams were inserted in the recorded pedigree at first probably for no other reason than because the growth of fraud and error necessitated some accurate method which would give a complete record and render an accurate reference not only possible but easy. Thus the correction of errors and detection of frauds and forgeries was greatly facilitated.

But, as so often happens with human inventions, the plan which was devised for one purpose produced a totally opposite result. The names of the cows once written in, the appearance of the pedigree left the impression on the eye that the cow was the superior element. This was greatly increased in America by the requirement that all animals bred in this country must trace to an imported cow. Thus the cow, and not the bull, gives the family name, and not only gives the name but controls the value of the family as well.

The accepted method of recording cattle pedigrees is nearly always misleading, and beginners cannot too early learn that if they wish to gain anything even remotely approaching a thorough knowledge of pedigrees and a facility in estimating their contents they must resort to the extended form. At the same time the abbreviated form is convenient and handy, and when once clearly comprehended is calculated to give a sufficient and immediate insight into the breeding of any animal. But to those who do not master the fundamental principles and familiarize themselves with the practical features of the pedigrees of the more frequently encountered families the record must always remain a mystery, and they will always be in danger of being victimized by ignorant or designing men.

Let us turn our attention now to some of the practical questions which meet us in regard to pedigree. In the first place the most important matter in regard to the pedigrees of all our improved breeds of cattle is to master the foundations of the most esteemed families. It is not so far back in the past since all our improved breeds came into great prominence as pedigreed cattle but that we may readily master the basal facts of their budding popularity and the way they became written into the records of each breed.

In accordance with what has just been said in regard to the bulls being chiefly esteemed in early times we find that as the breeds break into daylight they are heralded by some great sire or sires. Such among the Longhorns were Twopenny and D.; and so also we find the first years of the growing popularity of the Shorthorn Durham written chiefly in the names of bulls; of the Studley Bull, of Charge's Grey Bull, of James Brown's Red and White Bulls, of Mr. Richard Barker's Bull, and later, as the day fairly came brightening over the hills, of Hubback, and of his greater grandson Favorite (252). From these bulls were bred many cows and many bulls. The cows were rated chiefly as being the get of these bulls; the bulls chiefly as they displayed the capacity of their sires as breeding animals. The bulls of the elder day were thus succeeded in popular favor by their most worthy descendants, and it was not for several generations and at least two or three decades that the cows, which were themselves by the great sires and produced to others great calves, won for themselves renown as the fountain head of excellence. Indeed, in a great many instances the reputation of families which in later day parlance attaches chiefly to the cow at the head of the pedigree is, as far as the cow is concerned, posthumous, the applause in her day having been given to the bulls which had combined with so excellent a result. Thus as horsemen speak today of the value of a Hambletonian-Pilot Jr. cross or a Wilkes-Morgan combination, the early breeders spoke of a fusion of the blood of R. Alcock's Bull with that of Favorite or a Hubback-Punch cross. As time went on, however, the families became more and more defined. The first step in that direction was in the way of special esteem for the stock of certain breeders, such as the Collings. As they bred and sold many bulls the cows which they retained for their special use became more and more intimately connected with their reputation. Naturally their affections became fixed on certain specially good breeders among the females, and their produce, both male and female, especially the latter, were retained generation by generation. Thus while the bulls were diffusing the best blood of all the famous herds throughout the country a little body of cows was coming more and more to represent, not only in themselves but in their produce, the best work of these great breeders. Each generation seemed to have in an even greater degree the highest excellences embodied in them. So the female line gradually encroached upon the reputation of the male, and in some cases though an animal might show a large and dominant per cent of blood of one herd, yet he would not be esteemed as of that breeder's families unless it came by the direct, lineal, female side. Thus we saw that Baron Butterfly, though over 54 per cent Bates, was not reckoned as a Bates bull, but as a Towneley; and though having thirty-eight parts of Duchess in one hundred and twenty-eight he was not reckoned as a Duchess but as a Barmpton Rose, though having only a little over 3 per cent of Barmpton Rose or Towneley blood. We have an example of this special increase of value in the animals of one breeder reckoned along the female line, in the fact that though Mr. Bates owned and bred many animals of many families yet those who breed Bates cattle as a fancy hold that the seven families classed by the female side, which he retained to the close of his breeding career, represent in a peculiar way his work, and some go so far as to seek to exclude all others from their herds, or even from the category of "true Bates" cattle. In a less extreme way families are very widely reckoned according to the breeders and the foundation cows. Thus the family known as the "Cold Creams" in this country, from the imported cow Cold Cream 8th, is known in England most commonly as the Furbelow family of Sir Charles Knightley; though not infrequently even there spoken of as the Cold Cream family, from the cow of that name sold by Sir Charles Knightley to the Queen, and made by her the basis of a celebrated sub-family. So the Gwynne branch of the Princess tribe is nearly or quite as celebrated as the general family or any of the lines which have perpetuated the Princess name. In these cases the Furbelows might be said to have made their reputation more as being of the breeding of Sir Charles Knightley, while the sub-family as great prize-winners in the hands of the Queen made an independent position, which was exalted indeed by the superiority of their descent, but in turn honored and dignified it. The Princess family has the prestige of being probably the most ancient, in so far as records go, of all the Short-horn families; while the Gwynnes as a sub-family of special merit have added a new distinction to their glory of lineage.

It is not surprising, then, that in the direct female line should now be sought the special family character. Nevertheless, though it is so natural, it is very apt to prove a snare to catch the unwary. In the first place it distracts the mind from a careful estimate of every element in the pedigree to a single one. I have seen countless instances of poorly informed breeders valuing animals that were not even pure-bred in the most exalted way because they traced in the direct line to some celebrated cow. Few who have not had special dealing with pedigrees would imagine how common it is to find animals with a bad cross in the bulls near the top tracing to the most valuable families. This was at one time made easy by the fact that forgeries, loss of records, and similar defects abounded. In later years these matters are more carefully looked after and the records are kept pretty clean, but still many animals with one or two bad crosses half a dozen generations back are by no means uncommon. And by using a bull with a single remote cross running to the "American woods" on a herd of the most faultlessly-bred cows the whole of the produce under our existing theory in Short-horn circles would be reduced to grades. Thus the idea of family in its ordinary application is to be taken with great care and caution. It is not enough to know that a given animal traces to a good family in the direct female line. To get the real key to the situation we must take the standpoint of the early breeders, and taking up every bull see that all the bulls in all the pedigrees have pedigrees running to good families. This is tedious no doubt, but all good solid work is apt to be tedious; and it is not nearly so hard as to buy a few animals at large prices on the faith of the family name in the direct female line and wake up some fine morning to find that they are little better than grades. I have had the misfortune to have to break the news of this sort of thing to a great many unfortunates, and I think they would have been glad to have taken a great deal of pains to undo what was irreparable. At one time I used to get scores of letters in almost the same formula: "Mr. Blank says this pedigree is bad. What is the matter with it?" And nine out of ten showed at a glance what was the matter, and had a little study been given to the fundamental facts of pedigrees the unfortunate owners would not have made so much trouble for themselves. It is often a very small rock that wrecks a very noble ship.

The beginner must make up his mind to take up pedigree after pedigree and look up every bull by number, taking the top cross and going through each cross in each bull's pedigree; make up his mind to forget again and again what he looked up, for pedigrees are most difficult to remember; to be perplexed, discouraged, everything but deflected from his purpose. After many trials and tribulations he will discover some day that he does remember something, and may perhaps be saved from an unwise purchase by his knowledge. Then he will begin to see that such knowledge has a cash value. Then a great many think that because they know something they know it all. In a short time they will find that a little knowledge is a very dangerous thing. If they stop and do not prosecute their studies it were better for them that they had never learned anything. If, however, they press on, after a time the detection of the contents of pedigrees becomes almost a second nature, so familiar do certain landmarks become. And there is nothing so valuable to the breeder as a perfect mastery of the pedigrees of the breed he is devoted to. Few ever become masters of this department, and if one wishes to do so the study must be begun in early life. Young breeders will do well to remember that the moral value and the position given by such knowledge is greater even than the monetary value, but that the latter, in saving from unwise purchases and pointing the way to wise purchases, is far greater than most breeders suspect.

In conclusion, as an old breeder of long experience, who has seen many fashions come and go, I may perhaps be pardoned for adding a word here urging all breeders to beware of taking the view that pedigree is gauged by the paper exhibit. As the pedigree is merely the record of the animal's descent, and that descent is only worth preserving because the animals enumerated were of so great merit as to deserve being remembered on the theory of hereditary transmission of their qualities, so in adding cross after cross to our pedigrees we ought to remember that merit alone adds to the value of the pedigree, and each cross made with a bad animal is adding a minus quantity and detracting from the real value of the pedigree. For a time fashion and fancy may maintain this or that family in favor and price because of the way the pedigree reads (because excellence in the past has won reputation, in most cases), but if unworthy representatives are kept on an equal footing with good, by reason of such fancy, a day of reckoning will surely come. In that day the breeder will suffer.

But he will have deserved it, and we have no tears for him. But the breed will have suffered too, and I cannot sufficiently lament any act that tends to undo the noble labors of the wise men of old time, who formed the improved breeds by their genius and transmitted them to us as a sacred trust.

PART III.—THE PRACTICE.

INTRODUCTION TO THE PRACTICE OF BREEDING METHODS.

We have already seen that while all the various departments of the theory of breeding are properly reducible to a science, and that the body of laws which we have hitherto been engaged in investigating may be justly regarded as the framework of that systematized series of facts, that there is no less in the finished rules of application of these scientific laws to the daily practical work an art. An art useful in itself, honorable and noble in its end, lofty in its application. I do not deal in rhetoric; I claim in all soberness of spirit all these things for the art of cattle-breeding. I have already shown some grounds for my belief in its dignity. It is for me now merely to give some of the rules and to show the reasons for their existence.

The outline of this practical art may be drawn out under two heads: the choice of the material to work on and the treatment of it. And under the latter head we have three principal divisions: housing, feeding, and general care and attention; divisions more dependent, perhaps, on the logic of facts than of thought, but sufficiently accurate and exhaustive for our purpose. I confess to just a little dread of the pure theorist. The man who in his cozy study evolves a fine theory of farming and carries it out without regard to anything else except his faith in his own theory, and utterly unconscious of every other thing, rarely proves a successful agriculturist; were it not from a desire not to be uncharitable I would say never proves other than a failure. The late Henry Ward Beecher's humorous account of his experiences as an amateur farmer, in which he depicted his immense anticipations, his beautiful theories, his small returns and large deficit, is well known to most American farmers. We cannot too carefully avoid such a condition of things. It is a common accusation that is leveled at writers on agricultural topics that if you want to see a badly-managed farm visit that of some voluminous writer on the care of farms. Perhaps they may feel satisfied when they have retorted in the words of the old Baptist minister who was a pioneer preacher in the Western wilds and found it hard, in his own personal conduct, to reconcile precept and practice, and who constantly warned his flock: "Don't do as I do; do as I tell you to do." It is sometimes well to serve as a warning; but I am afraid that most writers of this class are regarded as warnings to others against writing rather than as against bad farming. If they warned against the latter and accentuated the evil by advertising it, they should assuredly be encouraged so far as possible to rush into print, for no lesson needs to be more widely taught and more thoroughly learned than that of the evil of slovenly, wasteful farm management

I am not going to try to inculcate, then, any hot-house, indoor theories; any fancies thin as air and tenuous as morning dreams; nor shall I seek to point a way which shall be only practicable to the few wealthy stock-breeders who can afford to use every appliance, however costly or difficult to obtain. Where the circumstances will admit of it we should seek to apply the strict economical law, that in order to rightly conduct any business we must have the most suitable material and the most perfectly adapted labor; that we must have the labor so utilized as to waste as little as possible of time and energy, and the materials so used as to get the utmost return in initial consumption, and also make use of the waste in some way to prevent its loss. But in many cases in Western farming we only roughly approximate this law, and I am too little of a theorist and too much of a practical farmer to think that the world is coming to an end in consequence. We must indeed work toward it. If we do not our boasted progressiveness is a delusion and a snare. But our conditions of life forbid our starting out with farms perfectly equipped with every time and labor-saving device which the ingenuity of the world has perfected. I look with a lenient eye on land wasted in this Western country, where land is abundant, by wide, sprawling worm fences; on water courses closely bordered by undergrowth of alders and sumac; and on many other similar cases of neglect; provided the land that is cultivated is *well* cultivated, the land that is cleared is kept *well* cleared, and the briars, and thistles, and burrs are kept out of every corner, and the whole aspect is one of constant growth toward complete mastery and utilization of every foot of land. "Haste makes waste," is an old saying, and in many senses a true one. It is better to waste a little land in using a sprawling fence than to waste more by missing the opportunity of good cultivation for a crop by consuming precious time in erecting a better fence. There is another old saying in England that it takes one generation to make a fortune but three to make a lawn. If this is true of a small plot of carefully tended land in an old country in which the soil has long been subdued and brought under the hand of man, how much allowance ought to be made for us here in the West, who but a few years ago began to reclaim a virgin forest from the native cane, and an untilled prairie from the wild and luxuriant growth of noxious weeds? We can afford to treat with an amused indifference the strictures of England's self-appointed prophet of "sweetness and light," the late Mr. Mathew Arnold, upon the crudity of our civilization, when we remember how nearly we have approximated in a few decades the work of a thousand years in England.

It is not for an ideal country, then, that I shall seek to offer some ideas on the subject of the practical management of farm stock, nor for some ideal state of cultivation and refinement in practice. I have been a hard-working, practical man all my days. I have had my ups and downs, my successes and my failures. From all, my failures, not less, nay more, than my successes, I have learned, and out of all these lessons I have drawn what I would fain call my experience. I say this dreading, lest others fear, as I often do, what men call their experience. How often do we confuse exceptional cases which take hold on our minds with the general tenor of our observation. It is so easy to remember striking instances; so hard to remember that the more striking an instance is the more extraordinary it is likely to be. And what we really want is the series of ordinary occurrences, not the extraordinary.

Our experience is of very little value if it is based on a series of judgments upon all the exceptional occurrences of a life-time. It may be very prosaic to talk of the thousand and one affairs of every-day life which are happening under everybody else's eyes as well as our own; it may be very prosaic, but what does it matter if it is? I am not engaged in writing a novel, but a practical book for practical men. It is a very prosaic thing. this raising of cattle, some men think. though Joaquin Miller has struck a truer key in his verse, which I heartily applaud, when he says:

> "And I have said, and I say it ever,
> As the years go on, and the world goes over,
> 'Twere better to be content and clever
> In tending of cattle and tossing of clover,
> In the grazing of cattle and the growing of grain,
> Than a strong man striving for fame and gain."

But despite the poet it is a prosaic thing to feed and bed down and milk and care for a lot of cows year in and year out; to have them fall sick always of the same old troubles; to have them grow old and die; life itself is prosaic. But also, as a true poet has said, "life is real, life is earnest."

> "Not enjoyment, and not sorrow,
> Is our destined end or way;
> But to act, that each tomorrow
> Finds us farther than today."

And I am sure that earnest men do not want fancy theories; they "want thought, true thoughts, good thoughts, thoughts fit to treasure up"; and more than this, they want the simple key which makes each thought able to unlock some hard fact of life. So I shall seek only to give out of the long experience which has been granted me such of the practical everyday facts and thoughts as I know or feel sure will be of active service to some—may they be many—of those who like myself are trying to fulfill in an earnest spirit the duties of our mutual calling. I am sure the indulgent reader will pardon the somewhat autobiographical tone of this chapter and those which follow; for I cannot speak in them with that decision which we may justly use where we are only expressing a concurrence in the conclusions of great thinkers and scholars; here I can only give my own views; they are only valuable as the observations of one worker in a great field. I do not state them as facts, but as what I have from my own limited observation concluded to be facts. I, indeed, am prepared to defend them and to maintain their truth and accuracy until I am convinced that I am wrong, but I cannot press them on others by the weight of any sanction such as we find in some other departments. I only offer the following pages as so many leaves out of my own life. They are the daily pencilings of nearly a half century of life in and about a stock farm.

SELECTION OF BREEDING ANIMALS.

It may seem unimportant to many to dwell upon this branch of our subject; they have already embarked on their venture and they wish only to know how to steer their bark into the desired haven—not how to build and fit and lade her. But I must differ with such a position. Beginners are often in search of advice on this subject and know not where to seek it. Others, too, who have made a more or less vigorous beginning are in doubt, oftentimes, of the wisdom of their start and need to be confirmed in the correctness of a wise step or warned against proceeding on a wrong path already entered upon. A very voluminous correspondence upon this single topic, extending over many years, has taught me how wide the interest in this matter is and particularly how many make bad beginnings and how fatal such beginnings are to after success.

I shall have particularly to do here with pure-bred cattle only, for I cannot for a moment think of advising anything so foreign to progress and thrift as that a breeder should set out with the poetic but unproductive scrub. Incidentally I shall urge upon the owner of that animal of ancient but unrecorded lineage the proper step to raise it into a new life and higher productiveness, but my subject essentially concerns itself only with the pure-bred animals of the recognized breeds.

The breed which any one determines upon is to be settled by his individual taste. I do not desire, writing as I hope I do, for more than the clientage of my own favorite breed—the Short-horn—to urge any one breed upon the rest of the world. I recognize the excellences—and they are many—possessed by all the improved breeds. If the breeder's object is the production of beef the Hereford, the Aberdeen-Angus, the Galloway, the Short-horn are all most admirable; for dairy cattle the Jersey and the kindred stocks of the other Channel Islands, the Holstein-Friesians, the Ayrshires, and the Short-horns all have their exclusive admirers; and they are not the only ones in each department which I might name for commendation, for the lists given are not meant to be at all exhaustive. There is, for instance, the valuable Devon breed, famous for draft purposes, and claiming to be equal to the Short-horn as a general-purpose animal; and also the Red Polled cattle, highly esteemed by some both in America and Europe. Any of these stocks offer good investments. The great expansion and large numbers of Short-horns would seem to witness to their supreme popularity; but I confess to looking on them with the eye with which a lover regards his mistress. While I have owned and bred other cattle, most of my experience has been gained from the breeding of Short-horns. Nevertheless most of the following pages have a general application; wherever the contrary is the case I will mark the particular application.

Having selected the kind of cattle which are to be bred, the next step is the selection of suitable individuals. This is no easy task in any case, and if the number is to be small and the amount of money to be expended in their purchase very limited the difficulty is much greater. Two things need to be very rigidly insisted upon, and unless they are the beginning will be altogether bad, and the result must of necessity be disappointing. The essentials of an improved breed which give it superior excellence beyond unimproved stock are individual merit and the guaranty, by virtue of long descent through other animals of like merit, that they will produce similarly good stock; that is, pedigree. Hence, individual merit and good pedigree are the two things to be looked for and insisted on in making purchases of breeding stock. Wanting either of these the stock should be rejected without a second thought. It does not matter how good the stock is, if the pedigree is deficient do not touch it; nor how admirable the pedigree, if the stock have not personal merit a good pedigree is the worst of delusions. The two things must go together. There is no middle ground; no room for compromise.

Nor is it difficult to find the right kind of stock among any of the well-recognized breeds. There are an abundance of cattle having the essentials insisted on. If this were not so they would not be slow in passing out of existence, or at least out of popularity. The excellence demanded is no fancy marking or series of markings; no white ear lobes, or feathered legs, or accurately defined markings, such as are valued among what are sometimes called "pet, or fancy stock," fowls, pigeons, etc. True some may reject a Short-horn bull because he has as much white on him as red, or a Hereford because the white face tends to extend into a white head; but these are things apart. The excellence really asked and insisted on is beef-making capacity in the Hereford—a frame formed for carrying flesh, filled out evenly and smoothly, and carrying most flesh where the most esteemed cuts come from, and with it showing the sturdy constitution which all healthy animals must have. In the Jersey, on the other hand, we expect the great, square, blocky form to yield to the smaller, lighter frame, wide behind, light in front; wedge shaped, as the phrase is; in fine, the typical shape of the milch cow, and with it the large udder and other evidences of milking quality—not insisting too much on a fine "escutcheon" unless we are quite sure that it is an infallible sign of milk productiveness and not simply a mere fancy point; and in the Short-horn we will look for all those evidences of the high-class beef beast which we sought in the Hereford, knowing that a Short-horn is first and before all else a beef producer; secondly, if we want a truly model Short-horn (and they are far from scarce) we will seek for one showing a large udder and other signs of milk production. The typical Short-horn should not be lacking here. Thus whatever variety of stock we fix upon we must acquaint ourselves with the recognized standard of the breed and seek to satisfy it in the animals we select. We would not demand milk production of an Angus nor a butter record of a Galloway, nor beefiness in a Jersey; but we must rigidly insist on having animals superior to ordinary stock in the special qualities for which we are adopting the breed; else, where would be the advantage in giving a larger price for a pure-bred than a scrub of equal merit could be purchased for? We have seen that the pedigree never promises good fruit from a bad stock, but the reverse; so there is no recourse to be found there. Having insisted on this conformity to the recognized standard in individual merit we must next apply the test of breeding and make trial of the pedigree.

A good pedigree is absolutely essential wherever a pure breed is to be bred. We have already examined into the theoretical value of pedigree. We now come to the practical question of how to apply the law of value. We must here lay down a general principle only. In every breed this question assumes a personal value, and in the jealousies and rivalries which grow out of this personal value the inquiries into excellence of pedigree become burning questions. But here we have nothing to do with fads and fancies; only with the general rule in its wide and ordinary application. Fancies rarely go very deep, though they may seem for a time to be quite strong and active. They are, indeed, like the breezes which ruffle the surface of the sea and make the white caps shine and gleam; that dash the water by the shore on high in sparkling spray, but do not after all greatly disturb the great body of water which sleeps in the depths of ocean, unstirred by the commotion.

In the first place a good pedigree is one which shows a series of good beasts recorded, one after the other, in the descent of the animal to which it belongs; and this being so it says: "Since like produces like, and all of these animals, all of personal excellence, have followed each other, each pair in turn producing an excellent offspring, ending at last in this meritorious animal, so this animal is in consequence hereby guaranteed to produce excellent descendants." This gives what we might call an excellent natural pedigree. In addition to this we must have a pedigree in all respects conformable to the artificial standard of the particular breed. This may or may not conform with the requirements of the herd books of each breed. We may say in general that most of the herd books are more indulgent than the public opinion among the breeders. Thus it is very well settled that to constitute a good Short-horn pedigree every animal in it must trace in every line to an undoubted English source, while there are many pedigrees in the American Short-horn Herd Book, especially in the earlier volumes, which trace to beasts whose history is unknown, and which goes out in this country. Such pedigrees are said to run to the "American woods," and this is quite universally regarded as a fatal blemish. We may say, then, that a pedigree to be a good pedigree must at least be conformable to the records of the standard book of registry; that is, it must either be recorded therein or only need to be offered for registry to be recorded. This is absolutely necessary. But many animals will be found which through some flaw, neglect, or error, though highly bred and of high merit, are not admissible for record. Are these to be passed over? Certainly. It may be unfortunate that such animals should be disqualified, but it is necessary to the purity of blood that all records should be strictly accurate, and men who neglect their cattle must suffer for it. The buyer should strictly avoid such cattle. There are many such in the country. I have spent many days of work trying to straighten out such pedigrees for friends who have sent them to me. Some have only been slightly neglected; others are hopelessly in the class of "lost records." But it is not enough for the buyer to avoid these; he must learn what pedigrees of those in the records are questionable, and avoid them also. There are some in connection with which forgeries have come to light; others—in early days a not uncommon class—have at the end of the pedigree proper —that is, after the last dam—the pedigree of her sire appended as if it were her pedigree, giving an apparently excellent pedigree to a cow that was really only a half-breed, at least so far as any record goes. When every sort of bad pedigree is sifted out then the residuum may be taken as good. But this sifting process is a slow and difficult one, and the requisite knowledge for it is only acquired after years of study. Then when this is done there are so many families left that every breeder naturally asks, Which of the good ones are best? So it is generally easier for the beginner to begin at the other end and learn of some one well versed in matters of pedigree what families are particularly esteemed and the grounds for their prominence. This may seem as if it were leaving too much to others; but this is inevitable. No beginner can without aid and instruction hope to master the subtleties of pedigree. It is a recondite science of which few, very few indeed, are masters. A man is very fortunate, and he must have been very studious, if he is, after ten or twelve years of active breeding, accompanied by constant study, possessed of a good working knowledge of pedigrees such as will insure him against making mistakes. The tyro must needs learn not merely from books—and there is nothing so colorless as a book of record—but from those more learned in the art than he, and to gain any working or practical mastery of the subject experience is absolutely indispensable. The beginner will generally find it the safest way to begin, therefore, to go to some old breeder of recognized knowledge and position, and of thorough reliability, and acting on his advice learn from him a first object lesson.

Is it, then, impossible to lay down any safe

practical rules for the guidance of the uninitiated? Yes, and no. A few rules of a general, common-sense sort may be given, but it will be seen that these are quite insufficient for practical guidance in all cases.

We have already seen what in a general way should be avoided. Now, naturally growing out of the fact that the two desiderata are individual merit and sound pedigree, we find that in any family the two things which lend prestige are extraordinary merit and ancient lineage. Thus in Short-horn families the Princess tribe holds a position of deserved eminence because it probably traces its recorded lineage to a more remote period than any other family; and of the different sub-families into which the Princess tribe has divided, the Gwynnes have won a prominent place on account of great individual merit. A few years ago in Short-horn circles the Loudon Duchesses were specially celebrated. Their then celebrity was due to the phenomenal excellence of the family and its success in the show-yard; but they added to this, descent from one of Mr. Mason's best stocks, and they commanded the approval of all on account of this. These are the two things to seek for. The seeker may by a little study acquaint himself with a few of the best old families, and make himself to a certain degree familiar with their history down to the present time and endeavor to find what he wishes in their number. But the utmost care will be necessary lest, some undesirable cross having crept in through the bulls which have been used on the good old stock, it should prove to have been in a greater or less degree injured. Too much care cannot be exercised on this point, and it is safe to say that with respect to most breeds no beginner has or can have the knowledge or skill to thoroughly examine and sift a long pedigree. The ramifications become endless, and the variety and miscellaneousness of the blood found in most animals so analyzed as to their breeding is astonishing, and the analyst inevitably finds himself at sea without a compass. Where all is blank to him a practiced eye finds signs and indications which tell him, almost at a glance, the contents of the pedigree, and he does not need to push very far along any pedigree before he finds a sure footing on familiar ground. If young and inexperienced breeders had more frequently in the past consulted honest and learned breeders before making their purchases there would not now be so many pitfalls for the unwary. As it is, many of our best old families have had so many bad crosses of all imaginable kinds put on them that only the most expert can be sure of sailing always in clear water. Many of these breeders have been deceived by designing men, more have sinned out of ignorance. Whatever the cause of their error its result remains the same—the practical ruin of their cattle.

It is evident, then, that nothing is to be taken for granted; everything must be based on careful investigation by those possessed of the requisite knowledge, and unless there is some one to whom the would-be purchaser can go to supply this knowledge and skill he is likely to suffer, or at least run a serious risk.

I have sometimes thought a plan could be devised, and would be eventually, though the time is doubtless not yet ripe for it, whereby the various societies of cattle-breeders would add to their record offices an office of certification, from which any one would be able to obtain for a small fee a certified copy of any given pedigree with a statement as to what it contained and as to whether it contained any errors or flaws or not. Such an office if well conducted could be made most valuable to the breeding public, and I am inclined to think that it could easily be made profitable. A few trained clerks would soon acquire great skill and would be able to dispatch business with great rapidity, and it would, moreover, be free from one of the great sources of expense in a record office—namely, the expenditures for printing. The value of such a department to the purchasing public would be great and immediate; and not less real, if somewhat more remote, would be the advantage which would accrue to the whole breeding interest, growing out of the rapid decrease of bad crosses put on valuable strains.

While I am no friend of mere fancy and no advocate of close family lines and monopolies, I am still of the most entire conviction that to breed cattle with success the cattle bred from must, so far as pedigree is concerned, be above the faintest breath of criticism. I of course do not mean as to comparisons, which the old proverb truly says, are odious; no stock can escape the negative criticism which comes from the ignorant or dishonest puffers who are forever going about and saying to their fellow breeders, "Oh! yes, your stock is very fair and tolerably well bred, but not highly or fashionably bred as mine is." There is always a certain class in every business, profession, and calling, who ignorantly, or knavishly, or boastfully set up themselves as possessing the only real thing. Some are honestly self-satisfied and complacently regard all they possess as better than that possessed by others; others do it "as one of the tricks of the trade," as they term it, knowing that silly men are to be found everywhere who do not distinguish the difference between notoriety and fame; between puffery and reputation. Such fancies and foolish notions run their day, bringing with them money and worldly success to some—indeed, much as a corner in wheat does—but eventually they fade away and leave the world almost unaffected by their advent and departure. I cannot advise anyone to run after such fancies. On the other hand, I would warn all to look carefully into the reason of the popularity of any special family or tribe, and to take nothing which does not show good quality and old lineage.

Some families of cattle are the victims of misrepresentation and malignance. Now and then in the history of competing fashions the owners of one family in the bitter spirit of partisan warfare have attacked the character of their rivals' cattle, and though sometimes unjustly and even falsely, the barb has stuck in the flesh. Out of such attacks, repeated over and over again by the malicious, the wiseacres eager to show a little knowledge, and the blind followers of these two more active classes, a fixed doubt has sometimes grown up making the stock sprung from these families bad investments although not badly bred. This is so for the simple reason that as a business principle no man can afford to deal in goods that a part of the natural customers of his trade regard with suspicion. I knew, for instance, a case many years ago of a gentleman who was rather free in expressing his opinion of pedigrees and sometimes criticised very severely those which were then quite popular. Some of his fellow breeders became very angry and assailed in very bitter words one of his most esteemed families, the members of which were of distinguished merit. He retorted that they were capable of standing on their own merits and rather defied criticism. Nevertheless, the evil name was echoed by many thoughtlessly, and by a few from envious rivalry, and in the end this old and esteemed stock of superb show cattle could hardly find a purchaser at any price; and though this was many years ago I suppose that family will never regain its former prestige in Central Kentucky, so long does the memory of such a thing linger and so sure is a slander to find an envious or a thoughtless tongue to catch its dying echo and send it forth on a new mission of cruel wrong. This is a good instance of the kind of stock a breeder must avoid with never-wearying watchfulness, and in order to keep out of danger from this source he must know something of the traditions of the breed he is purchasing as well as of the records.

It may be said that the very avoidance of such pedigrees tends to keep alive the prejudice against them. True, in a certain sense, and while I regard the words that Tennyson applies to the late Prince Albert when he says that he "spoke no slander; no, nor listened to it," as almost as high praise as can be given to man, yet one must never, as a business man, forget the fundamental law of self-preservation. If we do not look out for ourselves no one will look out for us. We may be pretty sure of that. And it is a poor kind of charity which buys the damaged goods of another at the price of sound ones because we do not want to hurt his feelings by letting him know that we have discovered the flaws which he doubtless knew all about. There is a golden mean in all things, a safe and honest middle ground, in which honest and upright principles do not yield to, but only apply, sound business sense. . We must inform ourselves thoroughly as to the character of the stock we are about to purchase, and finding flaws, unjustly attributed defects, or any other things that would make our purchases unproductive of profit, we must strictly keep away from them. We need not go away and tell everybody about them, nor even whisper them to the quiet night air; lest like the man who had in an unhappy moment learned that King Midas had the ears of an ass under an injunction of the deepest secrecy, could not contain it, and thinking to lift the burden from his heart without divulging it to the world whispered it to the reeds by the river bank, only to hear the reeds re-echoing and the winds laden with his whispered "King Midas has ass' ears." It is a true lesson taught by this old world fable that a secret intrusted to a light and vain mind might as well be spoken upon the housetop. Good sense and sound ethics alike condemn the injury resulting from gossiping about our neighbors' property to their hurt. We have only a right to investigate and make ourselves, so far as possible, cognizant of the entire history of cattle we are thinking of purchasing, and on the facts learned we may justly form our judgment and guide our conduct.

I am speaking here only of such matters as come under the head of prejudice. I think facts, properly speaking, ought as a rule to be open to public scrutiny. All questions of history are naturally of a public rather than a private nature, and should therefore be accessible to all. All questions of forgery, tampering with records, etc., are also public coñcern, and one who knowingly conceals such things in most cases makes himself *particeps criminis* by the very act. We are, however, going beyond the proper purview of our subject here. And yet it is of more importance to get these matters fairly before the mind of the new breeder than wouid appear upon the surface.

Let us return now with a little more particularity to the question of selection of the animals for personal qualities. We have looked at the question thus far in a broad and general way. We have seen that personal excellence and sound pedigree are absolute essentials. But there are very many animals having these qualities, so we must go to work to make specific rules for each particular case. Suppose we were to say that our chief end in selection would be to get the best we could find; the question would at once rise, What do you mean by "best"? Probably no two men are quite at one on this subject, and the herd if selected by several men might present a very heterogeneous character. Suppose we were to set out and find a nice little cow four years old, fully matured, round and plump in every part, neat in bone to a perfection, weighing 1.200 to 1.300 lbs., and carrying all she ever would likely carry in weight; and next a compact, good young cow of three years old, not yet settled in shape, and weighing 1,400 to 1.500 lbs.; and then a great, massive Scotch-bred cow five years old, and only just attaining maturity. low to the ground, tipping the beam at 2.000 lbs., and carrying it evenly and well; and then a neat, gay heifer of great style and carriage, a trifle long in the leg, a shade too flat in the ribs it may be, but with fine depth and admirable finish. Here are four quite typical Short-horns. Each sort has its admirers and its champions. In choosing our herd would we take in such animals without regard to anything but that all had merit and were good beasts? This is quite an important point, and worth something more than a cursory inquiry.

The real question put to us is: Is it desirable to have a special model, or is it rather preferable to breed in a general way for beef cattle, or for milk production, and so on? Now it is clear that among beef cattle there are many types. In some there is more substance, but often with coarser bone and more offal than in others. Some are fine in bone, gay, and stylish, but show a less vigorous constitution; and so on. In dairy cattle some animals produce large quantities of milk, but of an inferior quality; others produce milk of singular richness in butter fats. Are all these varieties to be mixed and mingled without regard to their peculiarities? Suppose we have such a lot of cows, the question is not far away what sort of bull are we going to use on them? The bull which will produce good results when crossed on one will just as likely as not fail on another —fail to "nick," as the saying is. This thing of a "nick," or a successful cross, is as difficult as determining beforehand how much an animal will inherit from one or the other of its parents. It is not the same thing, though at first sight it might seem to be. It is simply how will the two parents interfuse? Both might be excellent and transmit good qualities to their common offspring, but the produce might fail in that great essential of evenness, or balance. We want an animal to be "well balanced" throughout; not to be phenomenally good in one point and miserably bad in another. So this question of "nicking" becomes important, and we cannot say that because two animals are fine their offspring must needs be fine. This we are not at all justified in saying. Fineness is predicated of a certain balanced relation of parts. Our law gives us only similarity to parents. But can we not get a little nearer to the rationale of the matter than by dismissing it as a question only determinable by experiment? I think that while an absolute solution is out of all hope of attainment, in this as in all else where Nature's laws are carefully and intelligently observed, we may come to a useful approximation. How shall we naturally proceed toward such an approximation?

In the first place it is easily seen that where there is great diversity among cows, one bull, however good, can hardly be expected to breed evenly. A bull of remarkable prepotency may indeed do well in such circumstances, but even he would not do excellently well. If of a small, compact type, he would tend to decrease the size of the Scotch type alluded to above; while if of the latter sort he would introduce an element of later maturity into some of the other strains, and in some his own even character and ability to carry great flesh without coarseness would appear in that seriously undesirable form. It is sufficiently evident, then, that some kind of evenness is desirable in the herd if all the cows are to be bred to one bull.

But is there not some further advantage to be found in maintaining a single type? Such, at least, has been the view of all great breeders. We may well hesitate to pronounce upon the relative excellence of the many types found among the many breeds. It is always dangerous to dogmatize. We may follow our own inclinations, and see in one type a more attractive form than in some other which may win the preference from a brother breeder. But granting this, while we discover one type in its perfection more pleasing in our sight than any other, however perfect, nevertheless do we not often see animals of the esteemed type quite inferior to those of the other? I am sure all candid minds see and have felt the difficulty here. The result is that if we were to go to a cattle show or other place where a large concourse of cattle were to be seen and pick out the best ten head of any given breed, they would in most cases represent very different, and often almost opposite, types. How much more pleasing to the eye than such a group would be one such as we often see exhibited as the get of a single bull—very even and of singularly striking resemblance. If we are so blind as not to see the superior excellence of the best of other types to many, even most, of our favorite sort, we are in sad need of a visual cathartic. We ought always to recognize the good in other kinds, but it is very nearly certain that any breeder will achieve better results by taking ten or a dozen animals of one general type than by picking up helter skelter as many of the best animals as he can find without any special regard to each other.

All great breeders have had some ideal to which they have aimed to attain. That ideal was perhaps never illustrated in any single animal in their herd. Their herds gradually grew toward this ideal, and the average of the best of their cattle would perhaps more nearly represent it than any single animal. One would have the loin, another the crops and chine, yet another the brisket and shoulders of the desired beast; but no matchless queen would show from tip of horn to tail the noble symmetry that the breeder had made his dream all his days. In the herd of such an one we may therefore not unnaturally look for such variations as would seem under a wise and careful method of assimilation and modification to be leading to that high ideal. It is not in a herd in which all bulls and cows alike are already reduced to a nearly complete family type that we look for great breeding. Here good breeding may be done year in and year out; a well-fixed type may be produced and reproduced; but we want growth—not mere reproduction. We have had occasion already to notice that the conditions of this life demand a struggle toward progress even from stagnation, for otherwise decay will in a short time ensue. Wherever this very close resemblance is secured, too, it is almost always due to one of two causes: first, the overwhelming influence of a master mind—a rare, rare thing—and second, to close in-and-in or line breeding. In the first case the mind that built is pretty sure to be wise enough and able enough to maintain the partly perfected work and carry it on to an ever-increasing better point; and as we are not likely, any of us, to belong to this class we need not worry ourselves about it. As for myself I shall always be glad to learn of my fellow breeders without essaying to criticise or instruct them. In the second, if the theory of gradual decay resultant upon in-and-in and close line breeding be true there is more danger than advantage in beginning by a choice of a lot of animals, however closely of a common type, even of high excellence, if they are nearly related.

The idea seemingly intended to be developed by the great experimenters for our guidance is simply that a general standard should in practice be made as narrow and personal as possible. That is, if all animals within a certain standard of excellence be esteemed good, we should still try to form some clear and distinct idea of which among them are best, and to aim to reach that standard in practice without being distracted and drawn off by somebody else achieving remarkable success in producing his best. The choice which we will make in actual purchases will even then seem very unlike to that made by some who take one or another of the animals as a standard and compare the most unlike to it. The real thing is that to reach a desired type you must vary on every side a little, and by years of careful, thoughtful breeding gradually attain the object sought.

It is perhaps necessary to admit that many breeders do not really breed with a view to attain such an ideal, but are content to see no further than the stock before their eyes and to use what comes to their hands as best they may. This is only half true. Many of the breeders who most decidedly scout the idea of their having any theory or standard in breeding are the very ones most tied to their own idea and theory. This is nothing strange: it is human nature, pure and simple. Many more of us are possessed of capacity to act, and to act wisely, than to reason out the why and wherefore of such activity on our part. Those who claim to be mere common-sense breeders are the very ones most apt to have decided views as to what is a good animal, and most likely to be utterly opposed to having any other sort in their herds. If they, therefore, work along for years with the same lot of cattle it almost always happens that at the end of their breeding they have stamped their stock indellibly with the mark of their personal preference.

But some, especially young beginners, have little or no such preconceived ideas and no definite theory. For them the only safe course is to select as nearly as they are able a uniform general type, securing as high a degree of personal merit as may be possible. Almost every one will find a certain ingrained taste which will guide him, and he will need to satisfy that at the very outset; and it is of great value to every young man, in whatever walk of life, that his taste be formed on the best models. If one begins by forming his taste on a scrub model almost any thoroughbred will seem a miracle of art to him; while to another who begins with the best of thoroughbred breeds the other's wonder will be perhaps a sorry and very undesirable beast. Before any effort at fixing on an ideal is made, then, a close and intelligent study of the best results of the best art among the most successful breeders must be made.

SELECTION OF BREEDING ANIMALS.

(CONTINUED.)

In addition to the broad and general points of information in regard to the selection of our animals there are certain considerations of a more special character, which are of the first importance. Chief of these are the matters of physical nature which enter into every calculation in regard to the power and regularity of their reproductive nature. In examining these questions we must, in a certain sense, regard the animals just as we might a machine for the manufacture of a given fabric. It is of no consequence to the purchaser of a machine that it be made by this or that firm, or that it be called by this or that name, or bear this or that brand. The thing he wants to know is whether it is capable of doing the work which he wishes to have done. Of course when he has found that machines of a certain brand or made by a certain person do better work than any other he naturally wants to use that kind in future; so when a man has found that the cattle bred by one man give the best results he goes to that man when next he desires to purchase. But there are certain things that he wants to know in every case. A man may be assured by experience that the reaper of a certain manufacture is the best and yet not know whether a new cultivator from the same house will give satisfaction, even though he may be sure that so far as workmanship and materials go it will be of the best; and even among machines of one class some are better made than others. A man may do his best and yet not attain the same or equal results in all cases; so there are certain things which it always pays to take a good deal of pains to make sure of, and there are just such things to be looked to in selecting breeding animals.

In the first place, too careful inquiry cannot be made into the healthfulness of the individual and the family of which it comes. This is oftentimes not a mere matter of form. There is not a little of congenital disease in the best stock of our country, and this ought to be guarded against so far as possible. Such forms as consumption and other types of tuberculosis are especially to be guarded against, and are dangerous in that by using a bull when young with such an inherited taint in his blood we may infect a whole herd without his having shown any outward sign of the disease, which often does not develop for years, lying latent in the system. Such congenital diseases not only leave their mark on the animal by infecting the blood and causing the transmission of the trouble to the latest generations, but they also leave their mark on the animal's outward form, and so warn the observer to beware. The chief of these warnings is to be read in a narrow and contracted chest and other outward signs of insufficient room for the pulmonary organs. Secondary evidences are sometimes apparent in the dry, hard, and insufficient coats, which indicate a bad circulation. All such evidences of unthrift are to be looked for, and when found are to be carefully considered as plainly indicating a want of vigor in the animal. In general it may be said that the largest possible room is required wherever the vital organs are situated for their most healthy action. To speak briefly, then, the animal that shows a broad, deep chest with abundant floor room, giving a fine brisket, a wide chine and full crops, with the region back of the shoulder well filled out, running down well to the fore flank, and good barrel with finely-sprung ribs is the sort that every one takes as the model of strong and vigorous constitution, and that is the sort the breeder wants. Wherever the contrary is found there is almost sure to be an unthrifty animal. Not necessarily an unhealthy, but almost invariably an unthrifty animal. And while the one entails a direct loss the other deprives the purchaser of making any profit on the capital invested, which is nearly as bad. I always think that there is little or no profit in a beast with a contracted chest and that shows a tightness back of the shoulder. That constricted look, as if a surcingle had been tightly bound around the animal and had left a permanent impression, is one especially distasteful to me as indicating this want of thrift.

But much of this inquiry must needs be left to the good faith of the person from whom the purchase is made, unless some unusual channels of knowledge are open in the special case. If there are any reasons for fearing any of the more serious diseases being congenital in the family the quicker the animal in question is passed by the better.

But there are other things to be inquired into besides healthfulness. We have seen in the earlier part of this book that fecundity was as heritable as any other quality, and that infecundity tended to increase in transmission, and that all unhealthy conditions were of great danger as inclining to deepen the unfruitfulness, generation by generation, till the race went out in true infertility. There is no worse taint in the blood of animals when the object for which they are valued and cultivated is the reproduction of their kind. It behooves every one, then, who is about to purchase stock to make all possible investigation and be sure that the stock which he buys comes of fecund families. This is not so sure a thing as it would seem to some. It is too common to think of animals as always going on like machines—turning out their one calf every year with only rare accidents occurring to reduce this ratio of reproduction. The more highly bred the cattle are and the more artificial the conditions in which they are kept the more uncertain and irregular do they become as breeders, without the introduction of any such special disturbing cause as hereditary infecundity. With that reckoned in it is hard to tell how bad the case may become. And this is not by any means confined to the females. The inheritability of infecundity may pass into and along the male line quite as well as by the female, and not only may, but it does do so. This is too rarely taken account of. I should hesitate not a little before using at the head of my herd a bull which was the produce of a shy-breeding dam. That these things are so is the logical and inevitable consequence of the laws of inheritance already inquired into, and we may generally feel safe in tracing them to their logical conclusion. Some of us are rather afraid of deductions from the best settled of these laws, regarding as we rightly do most questions in breeding to be dependent upon facts of observation and inductions therefrom.

But why should we prolong the labors of investigation and work out each problem for itself when a sufficient number of particular cases have already been observed and accurate generalizations made upon them? It is the part of wisdom to act on the light thus at hand, taking advantage of what we have, and thus saving ourselves many trying and disastrous experiments. Nevertheless it seems to many as if it was placing a great deal of faith in mental processes to go to the extent of rejecting a lusty, well-formed, and active bull because his dam and grandam were very infecund. In most cases it will be found indeed that the bull does not show the lack of power to the same degree as would the females—certainly not to the same absolute extent. That were not to be expected; it is only in a proportionate degree, being as infecund as compared with a vigorous bull as a female when compared with a regular breeder, the practical outcome of which would be that the bull would prove increasingly uncertain as a breeder as he grew older, and gradually, at an early age, lose his potency. Sometimes this occurs without any one suspecting the cause, and not infrequently it is attributed to some other cause quite foreign to the true reason.

One need not remind breeders of dairy cattle how important it is not merely to ascertain, when possible, the capacity of the animals themselves, both for richness and quantity of milk, but also of their ancestry. This is a practical every-day matter that is too regularly looked after to be other than a matter of course. Here there is a convenient standard, the conformity to which may be readily tested. Both branches of the dairying business have reached a point in their development of tests of excellence which the owners of breeds kept for other purposes may envy but can hardly hope to imitate. There is no failure among these milk and butter producers to recognize the further fact that the bulls used on their cows must come from dairy families of merit in the line sought to be developed, whether butter or cheese production. In other words, they clearly recognize the principle that one sex holds in abeyance, but transmits to the descendants in the third generation, the secondary sexual qualities of its ancestor of the opposite sex.

These qualities are all, then, equally applicable to both sexes, and must be sought equally in each. There are besides certain qualities chiefly or solely applicable to the bull, and as the bull plays so large a part in the herd they are of the first importance. It becomes necessary, therefore, to take up somewhat in detail some of the important qualities to be sought in the bull to head the herd.

In the first place it is to be remembered that the bull represents fully one-half of the breeding ratio of the herd. He is one of the factors in every product, and he may be far more than half. If he is a vigorous animal of great prepotency it will not be long till it becomes apparent that he represents far more than his numerical value in the final sum of influence in determining the form and value of the results of breeding. This being so the greatest care and attention must be given to the selection of a breeding bull; care to avoid a poor animal and inferior breeder; care to select a fine animal and vigorous breeder; above all, to get a beast that will prove a superior breeder.

It is not an easy thing to find just the bull that fulfills such requirements. On the contrary, it is very difficult. Hence the more reason is there that every possible effort should be enlisted in so important and so difficult a task. If we are buying a young and untried animal the difficulties are only increased. Yet I am not seeking to discourage, only to warn and equip with the true spirit of trying many before choosing one. There is no point more essential to success than the careful selection of a sire. Let us see, then, what some of the more essential requirements are.

Following the general division of the subject into individual merit and excellence of pedigree, we see that if it is desirable that all our breeding cattle should have the utmost degree of personal excellence, in the bull it is pre-eminently necessary. It is possible that even the most fastidious might be willing, for one or another reason, to retain a cow of mediocre quality in the herd; but it is quite inconceivable that any wise or ordinarily well-informed man should be willing to breed to a bull of poor quality. It is nothing less than sowing the wind, and the reaping will surely be the whirlwind. Not only ought the bull to have merit of a high order, but it must be of a sort to commend him for breeding purposes. One of the essentials is what we call "masculine character." Just what is meant by this masculine character is difficult to explain, and the expression is often misapprehended. We may say that on the one hand, while it is by the very terminology of the phrase distinctly differentiated from anything approaching effeminacy—too delicate form and finish, or any of those indications of want of sexual vigor which are specially to be seen in the steer—it is never to be confounded with coarseness. It has nothing in common with coarseness. Big bones, awkward build, clumsiness, though sometimes mistaken for it, are in no sense masculinity. It is rather the air of active vigor, which is more in what we might call expression than in shape, were it not that it always goes with a strong, well-knit, close-compacted frame. The head in its bony frame-work is larger, the neck fuller and more arching, the body more widely set on the front legs than in the female; and then over it all plays the indescribable air, gay, aggressive, vigorous, which appeals at once to the eye, however hard it may be to portray with the pen. Such a bull will not be likely to "lose his personality" among the cows. Delicately-shaped, undersized, and too neatly finished bulls, and dull, stolid, inactive beasts are not desirable to breed from, nor are great, rough, coarse-boned bulls.

Among those qualities which are reckoned essential characteristics of the particular breed the breeding bull should want none, or where such excellence proves unattainable as few as possible should be lacking, and those of the smallest consideration. In most of our breeds those qualities which are regarded as really essential are few, and almost any animal that pretends to merit can exhibit them all. The only difficulty is to show them in a high degree of development. So regular are many of the breeds in reproduction that even this would be by no means a difficult task if more breeders would pay stricter attention to choosing bulls with a view to the cows to which they are to be bred. This often is quite important. A great rough bull put upon a herd of neat-boned, undersized cows will in more cases make ragged calves than good calves of an average size. Rapid transitions are not to be desired, nor can rapid and intensely radical changes be made except at serious risk. Where a herd has become undersized for any reason three or four generations are few enough for the work of increasing the size, and a medium-sized bull of a closely similar general type with the cows should be chosen for the first cross. Thus we find as a general rule we should choose not merely a fine bull but one whose type of excellence is closely akin to the cattle on which he is to be used. Not only so, but he should in addition be chosen with a view to improving the cows in some definite particular. I am always for progress. When we give up seeking to advance we are sure to begin a retrograde movement. In choosing a bull, therefore, we should first study our cows and analyze their defects and see where they are most deficient and where most easily improved, and then seek a sire calculated to raise up from them descendants far surpassing their dams. This is no visionary theory. None of us need fear lest his analysis will not bring to light, if honestly done, many faults and many flaws which the right kind of a bull would do much to improve. It is true that it is not always possible to find just the bull we want for the work, yet we very often can, and it is certainly worth the trial.

As the animal is to be used for breeding his power of transmitting to his descendants his own qualities becomes of the highest importance, and as that depends largely not only on his physical vigor but on his breeding also, we must consider the excellence of pedigree next in order. By excellence of pedigree I would indicate the greatest number of ancestors of the highest order of merit. The bull should not want here. The more animals of high quality from which he can trace his descent and the nearer they are to the top of the pedigree the greater is likely to be the bull's capacity for reproducing his inherited excellence. If this be not so then the whole idea of pedigree is a delusion and a snare. Pick your animal to breed from, then, not simply for his own merit, but look to see where he got that merit, whether from sire or dam or both, or from some more remote ancestor, and among rival claimants for favor choose the one whose sire and dam show most merit. This has a two-fold significance. In the first place, under the simple law of inheritance we have the rule that "like produces like," and the longer the type has been fixed—that is the larger the number of ancestors conforming to a given standard—the stronger and more invariable is this rule. Not only so, but in the second place a long fixed type of this sort exhibits a prepotent power over a less fixed type. Thus we saw that a highly-bred bull when bred to a scrub would almost surely govern and determine the nature of the produce. This is the extreme case; the variations are infinite to the point in which two equally well fixed types meet on an equal footing. Among these intermediate instances lie all those many cases in which a poorly-kept-up family yields to the greater vigor of a more vigorous family. Thus often in actual practice we find families bred for generations only for the purpose of keeping up some fancy theory of breeding whose paper results alone are definite, the animals meantime undergoing all kinds of vicissitudes. After a time they are crossed with a vigorous family bred only for individual merit and maintaining it and force of character generation after generation. At once a transformation results. The cross proves prepotent; the poor, abused, disorganized stocks yield to the spell of fresh and unpolluted blood and at once produce far better offspring than themselves or than their ancestors for generations. It is the final result of oft-repeated reproduction of a combination of qualities which gives prepotency, and prepotency is the greatest of possessions for a stock bull.

Nor do I speak rashly when I claim for excellence the power to reproduce excellence, and for oft-repeated excellence the power to deepen and quicken in all those having the double portion of excellence, personal and inherited, the power of transmitting it with increased force. There was a time when men looked more to the paper pedigree for in-and-in crosses and calculated that prepotency increased directly as these crosses increased. I believe that theory has in the main had its day. I am accustomed to look at the prize lists in England and America for the great proof of the inheritance of prize-winning qualities. Study the records of the great shows and you will be astonished to see how surely great prize-winning bulls send prize-winning calves and grandcalves to stand for them and witness to the permanence of their powers. Trace back the pedigree of the great prize-winners of today and their breeding is seen to be filled with the records of many a well-won field.

But this great power may be a two-edged sword. Prepotency may be for evil as well as for good, though naturally only valued when for good. But often an animal is a hopelessly bad breeder, getting the meanest calves from the finest cows. This is in the strictest accord with the law. But instead of being sought it must be avoided. I have seen the offspring of most excellent families indelibly stamped with the evil likeness of a deeply prepotent family with which they had been crossed. And as this inheritance extends to all things of form, of organ, of function, of health and of disease, how anxious should be the attention given to all these things. It looks almost as if the risk of a bad result was so great from an inferior but prepotent bull that it would be almost better policy to keep strictly to bulls of little or no prepotency, leaving it to each individual cow to determine the chief characteristics of her progeny. On the other hand, think of the transformation sure to be effected by a great sire of sturdy powers. The impress of such bulls as Goldfinder, the old Duke of Airdrie, and Muscatoon not only glorified the individual herds to which they belonged, but marked the local herds and even spread widely in the whole state and country.

It is evident, then, that sturdy constitutions are specially to be desired and the least symptoms of disease, or even feebleness of physique in the smallest matters, are to be stringently avoided. For in all breeding animals there is no consideration at all comparable to entire healthiness.

We must now notice further the relation of the pedigree to the artificial standard. What we have seen to apply to all in a general way applies to the herd bull in tenfold greater force.

For the least flaw in his pedigree will be at once communicated to all the produce of the herd. Like the circles formed by a pebble dropped into water, the evil goes on ever broadening. We must apply the pedigree rule, then, not in a broad and general way, seeking only good animals sprung from others equally good, but we must study all the requirements of such artificial standards as our various herd books, and let no flaw, judged by their standards, creep into our bull's breeding. Not only so, but we must inquire not merely of such standards but also if public opinion has narrowed their lines and confines to the narrowest limits. Even foolish fancies, where they are widespread, while we despise them, must not infrequently be recognized, and if not conformed to, at least regarded in so far as to avoid anything directly under their ban. This must be done, because in business we must keep in the front of the market or we will have a hard time. The principles we sacrifice, if we are called on to sacrifice any, are in no sense principles of honest dealing either in act or thought, but only in reality theories, which, however sound, must at times yield to the stern logic of events which is so eminently practical.

As to age, a vigorous young bull is more apt to give good results than an old and well-tried bull, because his purchase, though involving more of risk, yet gives the buyer the greatest period of usefulness—the vigorous days of early maturity. If judiciously managed a bull ought to retain his full vigor till ten years of age, and in some cases there is a manifest advantage in buying a thoroughly-tested bull, even though the price be proportionately high. There is then no risk of losing a whole year by having an inferior lot of calves come from a new bull which fails to reproduce his own good points; and the risk in many cases far exceeds the difference in price. But a really excellent breeding bull can rarely be purchased after he has made his mark. So that he who seeks a first-class bull must generally buy a calf and take the risk of his turning out well. Hence it is that one needs be so very judicious in the selection.

To sum up briefly, then, the stock bull should be of the highest possible merit, according to the most exacting standard of the breed, showing all those points which indicate constitutional vigor highly developed, healthy and sprung of healthful parents, highly bred, tracing through the best families, particularly those celebrated for producing animals of superior quality, in every respect conforming to the established and popular standards of breeding, and finally, where data exists for such a conclusion, exhibiting prepotency as a breeding animal. That sounds like a most formidable catalogue of requirements, but it contains nothing that is not of the most important nature. The breeder in actual practice lumps them all in a general way instead of drawing them out in a long analysis, but no practical man would think of foregoing one of them.

Thus far I have spoken of selection exclusively from the standpoint of the beginner, as offering the most logical method of discussion, and because the established breeder can readily apply to his particular case the principles laid down. Nevertheless, lest there should seem to be some lack of definiteness in this most important matter, a few words of special application may perhaps not be out of place.

The text for the fully established breeder is, Reject fearlessly all poor animals. If heroic pruning is good for the tree, the same policy is good for the herd. Let no unworthy animal be spared. Let the shambles have its own, and never run the risk of getting the average of the herd lowered. The mere moral effect of having a few mean animals in the herd is bad; bad on the owner by constantly lowering his standard of excellence, and worse on the purchasers who want as little to do with mean stock as possible. Weed out the herd, then, every year, on this account, but even more because the bad tree will inevitably yield evil fruit. The poor cattle will almost surely breed as bad or worse. Above all things do not keep a bull for service which does not come up to and surpass the standard of the herd. It is true it may be years at a time before a bull is bred, even on large farms, which in all things conforms to the highest standard, but when he does appear he is a treasure of the first value. In the meantime we often have to put up with animals of a lower grade, but not necessarily with any but truly fine and well-bred animals; and it should be a real necessity which is allowed to drive the breeder to accept anything but a bull of the very highest class. Unless the standard is placed and kept high there is no hope of true improvement, and there is an end, even, of successful breeding. A celebrated breeder of greyhounds is reported to have replied, when asked how he managed to breed so many dogs of such unusual excellence: "I breed many and hang many." In that answer was, indeed, the key to success. A very few out of many are to be retained for breeding purposes if the highest excellence is to be reached. Above all things learn to shun the delicate, unthrifty and weak in constitution. No animal, however fine, if of feeble constitution, can be expected to breed well, least of all can prepotent power be looked for in a bull of delicate health. And of course, where delicateness runs into positive disease, the danger of breeding from them increases in a rapid ratio.

Aside from these aggressive dangers there are tendencies to inferior usefulness exhibited by many animals which impair or destroy their usefulness in the herd and point them out as proper subjects for the pruning-knife. Thus we find among cows often those that are shy breeders, that are slow to come in heat after calving, that rarely stand till served several times, that occasionally lose their calves, and in the end show a very poor account of profit and loss. Others are never able to breed a calf as good as themselves and are a constant source of disappointment to their owners. So, too, with the bulls. How frequently do we hear of bulls being uncertain breeders. Few seem to realize how much actual loss comes to the breeder from an uncertain bull. In ten years' time almost a whole year will be lost; that is to say, one-tenth less calves will be produced in the herd. And yet men will go on using a bull which will rarely ever get a cow with calf at the first or even the second or third service. So some bulls are hopelessly bad breeders. Some very fine bulls which I have known have been simply miserable as breeders. Some men do not seem to grasp the fact that the bull is the cause of whole crops of mean calves, and will go on using him and speculate why their luck should be so bad. It is far from sure that a good bull will be a good breeder, though that is the natural and just presumption; but where the presumption fails the bull should be disposed of promptly.

There is a question often asked in this connection which demands some notice, namely: whether it is safe to breed from a bull of vicious temper. We have seen that peculiarities of temper and disposition were equally transmissible with bodily peculiarities and defects. The natural inference, therefore, would seem to be that it is dangerous to breed from a bad-tempered bull. The inference naturally derived from the theory is, however, to a certain degree negatived by my experience. I have never bred nor reared a bad or vicious bull. I have repeatedly bred cows to dangerous bulls and never had a dangerous or unruly calf. In this I speak exclusively of Durham or Short-horn cattle. I have noted, on the other hand, that a large proportion of the bulls of such smaller and more nervous breeds as the Jerseys were fractious. After long study and frequent discussion I have reached the conclusion that very much depends on two considerations: first, the general balance of the nervous temperament of the breed; and second, the method of treatment pursued from early calfhood; in fine, the education. In man the nervous, emotional and mental sides of his nature are most prominent, and are most developed by education and training. Social intercourse almost inevitably develops all the latent elements, and especially does the struggle for existence and the constant attrition of tempers among men tend to bring out all the irascibility natural to them. But among most animals the contrary is true. There are of course notable exceptions, of which the horse in his constant relations with man is most prominent; but most animals live a life under domestication the tendency of which is to make their existence a mere routine of eating and sleeping, and of this no class of animals are better examples than our cattle. And among cattle the beef breeds, with the tendency to great bulk and great flesh, the influence of which even among men is sedative, are particularly prominent for the placidity of their character. Excitable and violent tempers are utterly foreign to such natural constitutions, though it is perhaps true that all animals, including these, are capable of being aroused even to violent paroxysms of temper.

Temper and all mental states, however, are not simply inherent and inherited, but they are largely affected by habit; in other words, the natural quality is greatly increased by being called into frequent activity, and on the other hand largely weakened by never being exercised. Habit, either *pro* or *con*, then, is a large element in this matter of temper. Children with naturally outbreaking and violent tempers are often nearly cured of this serious moral disease under a mild and gentle regimen which affords no reason for its outbreak and suppresses the first signs of its rise by prompt action.

These two ideas are the basis of that treatment or training which seems, at least among the heavy and plethoric beef breeds, to suppress the disposition to temper, even when inherited: a life of perfect quiet, with full rations and abundant out-of-door exercise with such companionship as shall not excite to temper. This is best afforded by allowing the bull to run with the dry cows already in calf, though I quite as often supply it by turning the young bull calves from six months to a year old in with the old bull, which exercises a patriarchal oversight over them. But the most important element is the treatment received from the human attendants. This must begin at birth, must be frequent and regular, and always firm and kind. However kindly a bull's natural temper may be, however gentle his inherited disposition, brutal treatment will be very likely to arouse bad temper in him. On the other hand, quiet but firm and unintermitting care will in nearly all cases prevent a bull ever having an occasion to show temper. It is not to be supposed that temper will break out sporadically and totally unprovoked; that a bull is going to quit his quiet cud, which he is placidly meditating upon under the shade of some wide-branching tree on a fine summer's day, for the purpose of chasing a man passing through his paddock for mere love of mischief. It is only when he has learned by hard experience that man is his enemy that such things occur. In nearly all cases the first outbreak is due to harsh and unwise treatment, followed up by nervous, timid, and consequently nearly always unreasoningly violent treatment, which gradually leads to a constant state of open war. Another large class of cases spring from accidents due to playfulness on the part of the bull and foolish negligence on the part of his keeper. I remember one particular case which well illustrates the way these things come about. A young bull about a year old was being led to the sale-ring by a man who was not his usual keeper and who did not know that the animal was very playful, and had not sense enough to be careful with a stout youngster whose disposition he knew nothing about. He was in quite a hurry, and started off holding the halter loosely by the end and walking ahead of the bull, and dragging him whenever he seemed inclined to stop. The bull was gay and started in a trot. and the man. feeling the halter loose, hurried on without ever looking back. Another stable boy seeing this called to him to look out or the bull would run away with him and drag him. Just as he spoke the bull started off. got the rope wrapped about the man, knocked him off his feet. and after dragging him a little way made two or three playful passes at him with his budding horns, frightening and enraging the man, who became very violent. Help came in time to keep either party from doing any damage of a serious sort, and the bull being carefully watched and handled never offered afterwards the least violence to his keepers. A little violence on the part of the rescued keeper might have begun a life of dread and retaliation on the part of the bull.

Believing. then, that the temper of a bull is thus so largely dependent on keep and care, I am not inclined to say that it is dangerous and undesirable ever to breed to a vicious or bad-tempered bull. Though, of course, in some of the small breeds it is more likely that the temper is transmitted, but among them so few are other than dangerous that it would be almost impossible to follow such advice were it to be given. Nevertheless, other things being equal. I should always choose a gentle bull to breed to. Of course here I speak only as regards the descendants. As for keeping a bad bull, I consider nothing more dangerous and undesirable; I would never for a moment think of doing such a thing. It is a duty to ourselves, our servants, and the public, to be very careful how we harbor dangerous animals.

SHELTER.

The subject of shelter is fundamental in any discussion of the general care of cattle under domestication, and yet it is one of those subjects concerning which there has long been much difference of opinion—a difference which is not likely soon to be reconciled. The varying circumstances of highly-developed and newly-settled parts of our country, of mild and severe climates, which we have so closely connected by reason of the intimate connection between distant sections of the country secured by the railway and postal facilities of today, render this difference of opinion far more radical in appearance than it really is. It is quite natural that a Massachusetts farmer should have a different idea as to the amount and character of the shelter which stock need in winter from that entertained by a brother farmer in Kentucky, or even from that held by another in nearly the same latitude in Dakota. The relative nature of all such questions must be distinctly appreciated and the proper corrections made for differences in latitude and longitude.

There is another factor which makes a great deal of difference in our estimates of the requisite amount of shelter for cattle—the purpose for which the stock are kept. If they are market cattle in course of fattening for the shambles the great consideration is, How can they be kept and fattened so as to attain a maximum weight at a minimum cost?—this cost being resolvable into three elements: length of time which they are kept, amount and character of food which they consume, and value of land and buildings which they occupy while being fed. If, on the other hand, they are breeding cattle, there are other considerations of equal importance with that of maintaining the cattle in average condition, which is the most obvious and often the only consideration recognized by the owner. The general health of the animals has to be considered from the standpoint of securing from them the best calves at the least cost of drain on their systems; and secondly, of maintaining in the breed a maximum of vigor. This latter consideration is too often overlooked, and the former not infrequently. Let me illustrate.

Ease, comfort and luxury, it is now well understood among men, while in the first place conducing to produce a sense of content that has the specious appearance of the painless unconsciousness of body which is the concomitant of perfect health, nevertheless rapidly enervates and lead to a lassitude which invites disease.

Over-indulgence in a life of ease and freedom from exertion almost inevitably leads to a low condition of the system. This in breeding animals is scarcely less dangerous than a state of actual disease, for the young come into the world feeble weaklings, unworthy, too often incapable, of reproducing their kind. We must, then, always keep in mind the purpose for which breeding cattle are kept, and treat them in a way which shall make them strong and active, and not pamper them till they grow even less strong generation by generation, till at last they become profitless and effete.

It will readily be seen, then, that where one class are intended for a brief life of from two and a half to four years, and the one end of the owner is to push them to maturity and a certain market condition and weight, that the chief consideration he has to keep in mind is the constant healthy state of the animal. But the breeder has to consider the healthfulness of his animals not only today, but even more, the relation of their condition today to a healthy progeny in the future. All authorities agree, moreover, that the more artificial the life an animal leads the more unhealthful is its general tendency and the more special dangers are encountered, and consequently that the more closely a life of domestication can be made to conform to nature the more healthful it will be. Of course two of the great destructive agents in nature's economy are universally to be removed—the periodical scarcity of proper food and the assaults of natural foes. To these we may add the protection of the animal from the more violent extremes of the weather. A large proportion of animals in a state of nature fall victims to these causes. To secure for them immunity from them is consequently to give them greatly-increased opportunities for growth, long life, and reproduction, provided always that in removing one baleful influence we do not set another in motion. To avoid this it is necessary to leave the animal as far as may be free from unnatural interference after protecting it from active foes and supplying with a liberal hand its needs. This preserves the robust constitution, the active temperament, the highest bodily vigor—all qualities of the first importance among breeding animals.

Taking this broad proposition and applying it to questions of shelter we arrive at a general law which may be briefly summed up as follows: "stable the breeding stock as little as is consistent with health." How much this will be will depend on the climate of various places. As there is nothing more miserable to look upon than a herd of cattle shivering in a wet, cold storm in midwinter, with tails to the blast and heads bent woefully to the ground, so there is nothing which empties the food-trough or, in other words, which takes so much of the food the animal eats to make warmth and merely keep life going, as exposure. Too much of this will exhaust the animal's nature and burn out the life slowly, if not more rapidly in some active pulmonary disease. Nevertheless some degree of exposure is necessary to enable animals to face the vicissitudes of life, and the great question is how much? For my herd, here in Central Kentucky, experience has taught me that the dry cows can stand all weather except a half dozen very cold days in midwinter, not only without injury, but to their eminent advantage. From this outdoor life they gain in health and transmit to their offspring constitutions unimpaired, so that the young bulls are able to go out to the far West and compete with the sturdiest in ability to meet cold and storm. The pity that is moved by the miserable picture of discomfort presented by a herd of cows in a cold January rain is then not so truly pitiful as that which sees in it a necessary evil of life which brings advantage both to the enduring dam and her yet unborn progeny. But on the other hand, it is obvious that in Minnesota and equally high latitudes a constant and warm shelter will be needed for many months each year, the only important modification being that the period should be as short as possible.

I have spoken of this matter first because I think that the injury done to breeding cattle by too much pampering, especially in over-stabling, is both very great and very rarely commented on. I cannot too strongly accentuate the great importance of keeping stock in as nearly a state of nature as possible. If this were done there would be fewer weak, consumptive animals in the country. True, if this method of treatment were suddenly adopted many of the now enfeebled stock would probably succumb to the exposure; but would it be any great loss? In our manufactories of steam boilers, for instance, all the boilers are tested to see whether they will stand the strain which they must be subjected to; and, in the testing, not a few are found wanting. Is the world any worse off for the loss of the defective boilers? So I doubt if the world would be any worse off for the loss of some of the breeding stock which must be kept alive by a system of preservation in pink cotton packing.

But shelter is not only largely desirable but to a great extent absolutely necessary. For all young animals, except in midsummer, it is indispensable; for milking cows and for feeding stock equally so. It needs no more than the mere mention of the fact as to young stock to enforce the truth of it. As to milk cattle it is not so generally understood that cold, damp weather has an immediate effect on the yield of milk as it should be. The effect is usually attributed to the broad, general principle that food is first supplied to the support of life, and as one of the incidents of this support of life, to the supply of fuel to keep up the animal heat; and in consequence when the demand for fuel increases, the food which had been devoted to the formation of milk is deflected to the fuel supply. While this is true, it is, in addition, apparently true that a sudden change to a cold, wet day, or a sudden exposure, produces a more instantaneous and radical effect on the milk supply than is explicable on this theory. The cold seems to stop the secretion of milk to a large extent, somewhat as a chill often checks all the secretions of the organs of the body. Thus good authorities estimate the decrease of milk at once effected by exposure to a severe change of weather to be from twenty-five to forty per cent. This decrease seems, moreover, not to be checked by a corresponding and instantaneous increase of food; the effect of the increased food not being felt for some time after it is eaten owing to the comparatively slow process of assimilation.

While in the case of young stock, and to a minor degree also of old, one of the objects in affording shelter is to protect against the danger of illness and injury from frost bites and chills, its great importance in the management of cattle is due to the service it renders in reducing the amount of fuel needed by the stock, and consequently in reducing the amount of food consumed, the cost of keep, and the time needed for bringing an animal to maturity. This applies principally to all young stock and to beef cattle, but incidentally to all cattle as well. As an example of how much food must be used merely to keep up the animal heat which is mechanically supplied in the barn, the following experiment with sheep, which are, perhaps, the best protected against cold of all our domesticated animals, is very striking. The case is cited by Mr. Nesbit, and came under his immediate observation. A Dorsetshire farmer put thirty head of sheep under a warm shed, and at the same time he placed another lot of a like number, of the same weight and condition, in an open field, where they had no shelter of any kind. The two lots were fed in exactly the same way, on an unlimited ration of turnips with coarse fodder. The feeding was thus continued throughout the cold season, and at the end of that period the sheep being weighed, it appeared that the sheep which had been fed out of doors had gained one pound per head for each week during the experiment, while those under shelter had consumed less food and yet had gained no less than three pounds per head for each week of the same period.* The shelter thus represented, in addition to the saving of food, the amount of which is not accurately specified, a gain of sixty pounds per week on the thirty head, which certainly was sufficient to more than justify the erection of such a shed.

The value of shelter for stock being fed for market has, in addition, the element of keeping the cattle growing. Periods of stagnation are always more or less disadvantageous. Stock kept out of doors through the winter find it difficult to do more than merely maintain their full weight even on very liberal feed, while the same stock stabled nights, for half the time, would show a substantial gain, and if kept indoors all the time a still greater gain. For cattle intended for the block the margin of profit has grown so very small of late years that it is quite important to save all the time and all the food possible, and two and a half year old steers well sheltered and kept growing through the winters will in most cases pay better than almost any other class. And it is less important what sort of a barn steers are kept in than breeding stock, so long as their supply of pure fresh air is not cut off.

To return to breeding cattle, even where the

* Quoted by Prof. Stewart, in "Feeding Animals," p. 84.

stock run out all the year it is very desirable that they should have some sort of shelter against storms. If nothing more is afforded a thickly set wind-break of evergreens will give some protection against the worst wind storms with their penetrating cold. But it is far better to have, wherever possible, sheds open to the south in which the cattle can find refuge from rain and wind alike, and by huddling closely together keep warm enough for all ordinary occasions. These pasture shelters are not necessarily expensive and can be made to afford great comfort to the stock besides delaying the beginning of the winter housing and shortening its duration in the spring.

As to the proper form of cow stable or barn too many doctors have spoken, only to disagree, for me to venture to speak with anything approaching confidence or except in the most general terms. Very much depends upon the financial circumstances of the builder, and even more upon the kind of cattle to be housed, and the amount of cold they are to contend with. In the first place, under no circumstances ought the stable to be so close as to prevent thorough ventilation and the free entrance of an abundant supply of pure fresh air. Without these matters are carefully attended to the animals cannot thrive. Fresh, untainted air is one of the first conditions of sound bodily health.

Warmth is not inconsistent with pure air, though many seem to think that a building must needs be close and stuffy in order to be warm. It does, no doubt, require more attention and forethought to secure both, but the result more than repays the additional outlay. If the stock are to be housed in a basement, mainly or entirely under ground, in most cases the air is sure to be bad and the conditions for thrifty growth unfavorable. On the other hand, fresh air need not mean draughts. A warm room with a sharp cold draught blowing across it is a perfect death trap to man and beast, and the animals will be far healthier if allowed to run in the cold than if subjected to such conditions. But neither extreme is at all necessary, and almost any form of barn can be so constructed as to avoid these dangerous features.

The first class of considerations in regard to shelter, then, embrace: first, care lest too great an amount of shelter be given for the good of the animal, particularly in the case of breeding stock; secondly, the importance of shelter to milch cows and cattle in process of feeding for the market, and thirdly, the importance of fresh air and thorough ventilation to the cattle. These relate especially to the health or comfort of the animals. A second class of considerations present themselves based on the convenience of the farmer; but a passing notice only can be given to them.

The stable which I have found most satisfactory in this State is of very simple construction, and represents, perhaps, the minimum, while the elaborate barns so much used in New York and other colder climates represent the maximum, of stable warmth. The two ends in view in the construction of this stable are convenience in feeding and in removing manure; and as nothing elaborate or expensive, but only the most strictly practical materials and methods are used, it offers a fair model for those who wish a simple and inexpensive stable. It can be readily modified so as to give as much more warmth as may be deemed desirable. It consists of a double row of box-stalls, ten by twelve feet, each of which are fitted with two stanchions, so that they may be used for two animals if necessary. These stalls are separated by a passage-way six feet wide, and over the whole there is a loft for the storing of feed, which should be as high as the timbers readily attainable will allow, as the greater the height the greater the convenience in handling and storing the feed. In the passage-way there is a feed-car running on a wooden track, which can be made to travel from end to end of the stable with the feed, and the troughs being on the inside of the stalls the cattle are fed direct from the car. The feed is delivered to the car through an opening in the center of the stable directly above the track, either by means of a chute or by being simply dumped from above. The stalls all open out upon a drive-way formed by a continuation of the roof outward, which is further continued until it forms another row of low stalls, used for calves, which also open on this drive-way and are boxed in on the rear. The drive-ways are left open ordinarily in summer, but the ends are closed in the winter and in stormy weather by large doors, which effectually shut out storms and sufficiently close the building against cold. As stated, the stalls open on the drive-ways, which form great reservoirs of fresh air, and in order to take advantage of this a space of about eighteen inches is left in the doorway between the top of the door and the joist above. This insures ventilation—as the doors do not fit closely below—and avoids draughts. Even in warm weather these spaces afford quite sufficient fresh air for respiration even when the doors are kept closed for long periods together, and they are so arranged that by simply opening them for a few moments the bad air is quickly expelled and the fund of pure air thoroughly renewed. While no special effort is needed in Kentucky to make this building very tight, it can be made so with little trouble, as it has a comparatively small proportion of outside walls and few corners, and the grain and hay stored above act as a blanket without giving any of the stuffiness of a basement to the stalls below.

The floors of all the stalls are made of well-trodden clay, which is incomparably the best flooring for any kind of animal to stand on, at least in my judgment. They all slope slightly toward the drive-way and there is a small drain along the edge of the walls. This allows the liquid manure to drain away and be wasted, which is, perhaps, not economical and to be condemned; but in few places in the South and West has farm economy as yet progressed to a point at which manure is properly preserved. The cattle are bedded carefully with clean wheat or rye straw and the manure is removed the first thing each morning, being forked from the stalls to a cart in the drive-way and thence hauled away.

It is not always convenient to house all the stock in a single place, as some of the pastures may be distant from the barnyard, and then the risk in case of fire is very great when a large number are sheltered in a single stable. I have often, for these reasons, found that a number of box sheds in the different pastures formed very useful adjuncts to the large barns. These may be made of any number of stalls desired, and should always have a small loft above them to store grain and hay and other feed. A favorite form with me has three box-stalls, and is ten by thirty feet in dimension with a roof of a single slope, affording ample storage room above. This sort of shed in a lot where only young heifers or young bulls are kept is very convenient; and a single box-stall of a like nature in the lot in which service bulls are kept ensures them quiet and is very desirable.

GENERAL CARE OF CATTLE.

ALL practical breeders find that it is the little affairs of every-day life which really demand the most constant thoughtfulness and cause the greatest amount of perplexity. This is natural enough, the more so that in a large degree these things can only be learned by experience. Assuming this to be so, not only in a large degree, but *absolutely*, those who have taken the pains to supply manuals for the aid of the perplexed among agriculturists have almost entirely neglected the subject of the practical care of cattle. This is certainly to be regretted, and the omission needs to be supplied. That this will prove difficult is beyond question. That it is, therefore, the better worth attempting is equally certain. I shall, then, in a running comment endeavor to give such practical hints as may perhaps prove of assistance at least to the young and inexperienced breeder. There are many points of view from which this subject might be approached, and an analysis from each of these standpoints would demand a different method of treatment. It has seemed to me to be most simple and rational to adopt the view which looks at the development of method along the animal's individual growth, and makes the discussion of the methods to be used follow the evolution of the animal's life history. This will bring before us all the questions affecting the physical side of the animal, either directly or indirectly, and while such questions as those of shelter, feeding, and so forth, demand a more exhaustive treatment by themselves than can be given in such a general discussion as is attempted in this chapter, they will nevertheless require some mention here, thus entailing a certain amount of repetition; yet such repetition will be from the nature of the case illustrative, and may perhaps be pardoned for this reason and for the occasional advantage which practical points gain by the accentuation arising out of such reiteration.

CALVES.

We cannot begin our care of the individual animals too soon. The demand for attention begins not only at birth, but rather some hours at least before birth actually takes place, in order that it may be carefully provided that the dam comes to calving in a safe and suitable place. This event of entry into even so cold a world as this of ours is no doubt a highly important—what men call an "epoch-making"—event to the youngster so informally ushered in; and it is scarcely less so to the owner. Every provision should be made for a safe arrival and warm reception. Especially in cold and stormy weather is this necessary, and when the dam's labor is long and difficult. In some such cases it requires not infrequently considerable persuasion to get the little stranger to actively assume the duties of life. In all such cases the cow should be put in a warm, sheltered spot, or if this should be neglected, it should be done as soon as the calf is dropped. In warm and fair weather this is of course unnecessary: my experience in this, as in all else, being that the more natural and inartificial the life the cattle lead, the better they thrive. Under all circumstances it is important to see that the calf is properly dried. In bad weather unless this is done a chill, which may result seriously, will almost always occur. Nature has provided her method for this, and the cow will in almost every case do her duty and lick her produce dry. But should she fail to do this, as sometimes occurs, especially in the case of young heifers with their first calves, the calf must be looked after. In almost every case it is only necessary to attract the dam's attention to her offspring, when, the maternal instinct being thereby awakened, she will do her duty. Oftentimes it is only necessary to place the calf where she will see it. Sometimes a little meal or bran sprinkled over the calf laid in front of the mother will be the best method, as the cow will begin to lick off the meal, and once started the maternal impulse is rarely insufficient. In some cases, chiefly where the cow is seriously or fatally affected by calving, artificial means must be used, which in such instances cannot be applied too promptly. This licking of the calf seems to serve not only to dry the calf, which in inclement weather is highly essential to prevent chilling, but also to warm and quicken the as yet feeble circulation, which as soon as the genial warmth spreads through the members leaps into full course.

When the calf has been thoroughly dried and the cow has had an hour of quiet the next thing is to see that the calf is suckled. This should never be neglected. While some calves are strong enough to get on their feet and suck for themselves many cannot do so, and it never pays to take any chances. Wherever the labor has been tedious and the cow restless the calf is apt to show the results of it, and where labor has been greatly prolonged it may not recover its full strength for several days. These calves must be held up to suck, and if they do not suck well at the first trial, frequent opportunities must be given. Unless this is done many valuable calves will be sacrificed at the outset. A strong calf which meets with no adverse circumstances in the birth-throes of his dam rarely needs any special attention after he has once had a good tug at his mother's teats, and thenceforth can take care of his own food supplies if only given free access to his dam; and it is very important that this free access should be given. "The child is father to the man" is one of the most hackneyed of all popular sayings: and the very fact that it is so hackneyed is the best evidence of the general approval which all men give to the sentiment which it embodies. So true is it that it not only applies to man but to all nature. "As the twig is bent so will the tree incline," is its exact analogue in the vegetable kingdom. In fine, as the young animal or plant is treated the mature organism will be moulded. The young animal that is placed in our hands may be said to contain *in potential* all the qualities of the mature animal. These qualities may be fostered and developed, or they may be stunted, hindered in their expansion, even atrophied by neglect. It becomes a question, then, at the very outset, whether the calf is the main consideration with the breeder, or whether there is some ulterior consideration more important to him which shall dominate and control his treatment of the calf. If the calf gets all the milk he can drink straight from his dam, and his dam is a good milker, the chances are he will thrive and grow and do well. Unless this is the case the chances are against him. If a little cream or butter is of more concern to the owner than the highest good of a valuable calf, of course then the calf must get on as best he may on some substitute for mother's milk; but if there is anything which really takes its place I have never seen it. If possible, then, let the calves have free and full access to their "base of supplies."

The calf is perhaps best off if allowed to have free run with his dam for some months. Its delicate stomach is best suited by frequent draughts of small quantities of milk. The cow, on the other hand, is apt to be a better milker if habituated to less frequent and more perfect milkings of all the milk in her bag that she can be made to "let down." Where interests thus conflict a compromise which will do as nearly as possible the most even-handed justice to all is demanded. My system has long been to allow the calf to run with the cow for three or four weeks and then to separate them, and from that time till it is about three months old the calf is suckled three times a day—morning, noon, and night—being allowed the first demand on the milk supply, the cow being stripped after the calf has had its fill. When the calf is three months old the noon suckling is discontinued and the other two kept up ordinarily till it has reached the age of six months, which is the usual age for weaning, although in a few exceptional cases the weaning may be advantageously delayed a little beyond that age.

Earlier than six months I am quite sure it is unwise to wean calves intended for breeding purposes. Milk is the natural diet and they thrive on it better than on anything else, and not till the calves are fully of that age are they able to do thoroughly well without it and to thrive on solid food. The weaning time is in a great degree a crisis in the calf's life. If cut off from nature's diet too early bad results not infrequently ensue; but if allowed to go on to that period at which in the natural sequence of events the calf would find his milk ration more and more insufficient and his capacity to eat more and more perfect everyday, the transition, instead of being violent, is at once natural and easy, and therefore without injurious consequences. The great thing is to keep the growth of the calf from suffering any check. If this growth goes right along all is well. If, however, the weaning is followed by a period of pining and real need of the milk diet, and the calf is for a few weeks unthrifty, the effect will be apparent in the animal's after-life, for these short periods of retardation in early life count up largely in the sum. This is not an easy matter to impress upon many men, and yet an animal that has an unbroken calfhood of thrifty growth will mature earlier and develop more completely the possibilities of its nature than another which, with equal promise, was suffered to get again and again out of condition by unwise saving in the first months of its life. Even six-months-old calves cannot always be taken off of their milk, although the utmost care be used, without showing the effects of it in a bad way, which is certainly excellent evidence of the very high character of this diet for the calf. What has just been said, of course, involves to a certain extent a condemnation of a skim-milk ration. I must deprecate the substitution of such a ration for the milk direct from the teats wherever it is not an absolute necessity. I can but regard it as a poor policy which sacrifices the best good of a valuable calf at the most critical time in its life to the securing of a little cream or butter. A little retarding of the growth at this period may mean the difference between being able to make a sale and not being able to do so. To command the market the best cattle are necessary. But at the same time no doubt there are occasions when this sacrifice is, or seems to be, demanded, and in all such cases the best that can be done is to yield to the apparent necessity and find the best substitute. It must be distinctly borne in mind, however, that a calf cannot thoroughly thrive on skim-milk alone; it is not in technical parlance a "complete ration": that is to say, it does not contain in proper proportion all those elements which are necessary for the growth and maintenance of a healthy animal. When skim-milk is fed, therefore, something must be added to it to complete its food elements. The most approved addition to it for very young calves is a little oil-meal. This adds the "carbo-hydrates" and other muscle-forming ingredients which are highly necessary, especially to the young animal; the oil which it contains acts as a laxative, also, and overcomes in a safe manner the tendency of skim-milk to induce constipation. Wherever it is used it is further highly desirable to press on the work of teaching the calves to eat freely.

Prof. Elliott W. Stewart in his valuable work on "Feeding Animals" says: "Fresh milk is the best food for the young calf, and the natural method of taking it is for the calf to draw it from the udder of its dam." But he goes on to say that where this is found impracticable skim-milk may be used, and "the ration may be made about as nutritious as the new milk by adding to it flaxseed gruel, made by boiling a pint of flaxseed and a pint of oil-meal in ten to twelve quarts of water, or flaxseed alone in six times its bulk of water. Mix this one to three parts with skim-milk; feed blood warm." No doubt good results have been and are constantly being secured by feeding such a ration, but I cannot give up the good old-fashioned way without a protest, and I would urge, especially on the breeders of blooded cattle, the maintenance of the time-honored custom.

In any case the calves should be taught to eat as early as possible, for it is important to supplement the milk ration both in quantity and in variety as soon as practicable. By the time the calves are two months old they will nibble at the grass in the fields and pick at hay which can be conveniently reached; and very soon after that age they will begin to eat a little corn-meal and bran very readily. When once they have fairly begun to eat they make rapid progress. By the time they are three months old they should have two regular feeds of dry food. Corn-meal is a good thing to begin on, and the daily feeds should consist of as much as they will eat up clean. As they progress both quantity and variety should increase; bran and oats, chopped hay, and any green food or roots usually fed, that may be available. It is generally a safe rule to feed the calves, both before and after weaning, all the food they will eat; but it should be carefully looked to that they do eat all that is given them and that none remains in the troughs and feed-boxes to grow sour, when cooked or other food that is likely to ferment is being fed. A careful watch must be kept over the calves, too, especially where their dams are large milkers, and at the first symptoms of scouring the amount of food should be reduced. In young calves this will generally be caused by an over-abundant supply of milk; in older calves by too much green food. The cause is generally easily detected and should be removed at once. It rarely takes more than a few days of quiet and reduced rations, or of dry and cooling, in lieu of heating, food, to correct these disorders of the bowels. Of course such troubles are chiefly experienced in the hot summer months or the days of lassitude in the early spring.

After the calves have been weaned they are past the first epoch in their lives, and may be regarded as out of the period of special care; nevertheless during the whole course of growth and development the feeder's attention should not lag for an instant. During all this period every effort should be made to bring out all there is in the animals. The feeder for market has learned how large is the return on beef cattle for liberal feeding in early life. This is a lesson the feeder of breeding cattle needs to learn far more thoroughly than he has hitherto. Many animals which possessed admirable possibilities have had their growth and development so checked by scanty rations at this critical period that they have grown up stunted and half-starved beasts. Two full feeds a day of the most nutritious food should be given both male and female, and every provision for good, healthy growth should be supplied. Among the provisions which I esteem as essential are an abundance of clean and wholesome water. There is no more important condition of healthful life than a suitable water supply, and there is probably no condition more generally neglected. Cattle often show strange preferences, speaking from a human standpoint, as to their water. Thus they will frequently cross a running stream, a creek, or a spring branch to drink out of a pond of standing water. This is doubtless due to their preferring the higher temperature of the pond water to the cold water of the stream. This naturally leads to the conclusion that very cold water is not desirable for stock. This conclusion is further supported by the well-settled physiological fact that cold water in any large quantity is injurious to the digestive processes, retarding, and if the chill occasioned by it is great, temporarily stopping them. Hence as far as possible the water given the stock should not be very cold.

Another provision which needs to be insisted on is abundance of out-of-door life. This is important for two reasons: First, because exercise is a positive condition of health in all higher animals; and second, because the close air and the restricted space of stables are exceedingly injurious to animals. With very small calves dropped in midwinter constant stabling is no doubt for a time an absolute necessity. They ought not to be unnecessarily exposed to the inclemency of the weather, but as soon as they can safely be out of doors they should have a daily outing, sufficient for exercise and for the acquisition of a sturdy constitution. As for summer calves there is rarely any need for them to be stabled at all till they are large enough to be put up for a part of each day to be fed, which I find the most profitable way to feed them. They should have ready access to a grass lot, which should be clean and free from mud, and large enough to afford good opportunity for healthful exercise, and not a mere pen. There should be besides an abundance of shade to protect the calves in the hot summer days from the direct rays of the sun.

Just how much out-door life shall be given the calves must depend on circumstances. It should be kept in mind, however, that the laws of nature should never be violated except for some good and sufficient reason. As the natural condition of cattle is one of unrestrained out-of-door life, the aim of the breeder should be to approximate this as nearly as may be. Of course in the excessive cold winters of the

Northern sections of this country this is not to be followed absolutely, for the cattle were not originally subject to such excessive cold, and would not thrive or prove profitable if exposed to it, but would suffer greatly and in many cases perish from exposure. Where man has modified the surroundings by transportation or other means he must adapt the other conditions of life to meet these changes. Hence in many cases continued stabling through the whole winter is necessary, and in others for the winter nights. These modifications are naturally yielded to as imperative. But stabling is often carried much farther than is absolutely necessary: much farther than is good, I fear, for the constitution of the animals. I seek to have the animals out of doors at least half the time. In the day-time in winter of course, and at night in summer when it is cooler in the pastures and the stock are not troubled, as they often are in the day-time, with flies. If the stables are close and hot of course it is open for consideration whether the caives are not better off in a shady pasture with an abundance of water near at hand than in the stables. Unless there is some special reason for it I do not ordinarily stable the calves at all in the warm months. But if they are being prepared for the autumn fairs they must be put in condition and their coats attended to, and this practically necessitates stabling them during the day. If the stables are very hot the calves will not thrive and a compromise may be made by putting them in any convenient shed which is capable of giving shelter from the sun and a circulation of air. The open air and plenty of exercise I regard as one of the prime factors in making thrifty, vigorous animals.

As the calves approach a year old those that are the best feeders will begin to take on too much flesh for a good breeding condition on the liberal feeding herein advocated. This is especially true of the heifers. As soon as this appears to be the case they should be fed only once a day if on good pasture, or if confined principally or entirely to in-door feeding the supply should be gradually reduced to such an amount as will keep up strong, steady growth without causing too much fat-production. The young animals want solid growth, bone, muscle and general lean meat-production at this period, without the addition of any surplus flesh. The heifers need to be watched with special care as they grow to be from fifteen to eighteen months old and approach the time when they are to be bred. It is particularly desirable that they should come to this time in as natural a physical condition as possible. Obesity, overheated state of the blood from an excessive corn diet or an over-supply of other heating food, and other similar unhealthy states are very apt to make the heifers shy or uncertain breeders, and very difficult to get with calf. With the young bulls the case is somewhat different, for while it is not desirable to have them in high flesh they must be kept growing vigorously, and if they are used early they will demand rather more food after they are put to service than before. Hence at the time that young heifers are being cut down in ration the bulls between one and two years will very likely need to be fed a little more. High-fleshed heifers, where they have good pasturage, will often be better off if not fed at all in addition to their grazing; but young bulls in order to retain the highest vigor must be regularly fed on grain.

One of the questions which thrusts itself upon us in regard to young stock is as to the wisdom or unwisdom of fitting them for the fairs. To speak in broad and general terms I regard obesity as always an evil and often a serious danger; and our fairs in nearly all cases seem to demand a high condition of flesh, amounting in most cases to obesity, as a condition of success: yet it must be admitted that under a year old there is little serious risk in preparing stock for the show-ring. Yearlings fall into a very different category, and as they are in the most critical epoch, especially for the females, the greatest care and prudence is demanded. It must be kept in view that overflesh very readily runs into disease, and that fatty degeneration is more apt to attack the reproductive organs than any other part of the animal organism. As the animals which it is desired to fit for the show-ring are sure to be those of the highest personal merit, they are, therefore, the very ones most valuable for breeding, and the very last ones which ought to be subjected to the perils of a show-yard training and feeding. I feel sure that even where many go through the ordeal successfully, that the most desirable breeding animals are those which have never been overfed, and whose systems have never been put to a strain by the application of any unnatural methods; those, in fine, which have gone on year in and year out in the even tenor of their way, living in peace and plenty in all seasons, and reproducing themselves annually with credit. Such beasts, I am confident, breed better and breed longer than those which are treated to long periods of excessive feeding for the show-ring.

The calves are decidedly better for being kept apart from the older cattle. I think as a general rule, that cattle of the same age or condition do best when kept to themselves. This applies with especial force to the young stock. There is thus much less risk of accidents and injuries than when cattle of all ages are herded together. Of course, too, the young bulls—at from three to four months old, as soon as they begin to worry themselves and fret the heifers—must be put in a lot by themselves. Otherwise they will not grow and thrive as well, nor will they allow the heifers to do as well, as when both are in quiet pastures living a life as free from disturbances and excitements as it is possible to make it. The run of the young bulls should be well removed and secluded so that they may not be in sight, smell or hearing of cows and heifers in heat, for if they are they will fret and chafe themselves and lose instead of gaining in flesh.

These provisions for the general good of the stock have also a commercial advantage which is worth noticing. There is nothing which plays a greater part in the sale of pure-bred animals than the mere captivation of the eye. This, indeed, goes further than mere blooded stock sales, but it is especially notable in regard to them. A prospective purchaser going into an enclosure containing animals of all ages and conditions, old and young, mature and immature, thin and fat, is confused; his eye wanders aimlessly, and unless he has a far better trained eye than most men possess he will get but a vague and indefinite idea of the cattle inspected. But if the calves are in one enclosure, the young bulls in another, the yearling heifers in a third, the two-year-olds in a fourth, and so on through the dry and milking cows, etc., each class speaks for itself. The impression is one of symmetry and congruity. If the purchaser is in search of yearling heifers his mind is not distracted by the superior impression made by the greater maturity of two-year-olds ready to calve which stand alongside. All who have dealt in market cattle know the superior selling qualities of a very even bunch of cattle. It is much the same principle here, except that the element of beauty of form is of far higher—almost of the highest—importance in the case of blooded stock.

For the best results in raising young stock I have already said that it is highly important to keep them as quiet and as far removed from excitement of every sort as possible. In order to secure this the animals must be handled systematically from birth, habituated to the presence of man—made to regard him as a purely beneficent being. Gentleness is almost a *sine qua non* of thrift. An animal that is being frightened constantly, that will bolt out of the stall leaving a half-emptied feed box behind it at the least approach of man, that will race around the pasture whenever an attempt is made to drive it up to feed or for any other purpose, is not likely to yield satisfactory results. They should be familiarly handled from birth, and always with gentleness coupled with firmness. The bull calves should especially be dealt with in the most careful way, never being struck or kicked and handled only in the kindest way. There need never be any trouble with an animal that is begun with early enough and dealt with kindly and firmly. Every calf should be thoroughly halter-broken before it is strong enough to make any serious resistance, and taught thus early that the process is one which involves nothing either of pain or discomfort, but is a mere concomitant of every-day life. Then when a calf is sold, or is to be exhibited, it will not require half a dozen men and a "battle royal" to get the calf to go anywhere. All of which means that the calf is neither contrary nor stubborn but utterly ignorant of what it is wanted to do, and too frightened to know how to do anything but make wild and totally blind efforts to escape. Instead of the calf being to blame it is the owner who has neglected its proper training and entailed on it and himself this wild and senseless struggle. Submission is a matter of education and may be carried to any point that the owner may desire, provided that he begins early enough and proceeds with sufficient firmness and method. And the more absolute the submission on the part of the animal the smaller the amount of friction and the better the results throughout the animal's life. Many an accident happens because calves are not properly broken to lead; many a young bull's temper is spoiled; many a young heifer loses her calf because she will not submit to the necessary human aid in securing a successful deliverance. Reckless methods, driving with stick and stone, are utterly to be condemned, and constant handling and the most familiar intercourse between man and beast is the one and only policy which leads to success. If I take my seat in the lot where my young heifers have their grazing they will gather around me, and push each other aside for the friendly scratch on the back which they expect, and if they do not get it will sometimes rub up against me. This is the sort of terms which in my judgment should exist between master and brute.

HEIFERS.

The word heifer is a somewhat indefinite expression, being defined by the dictionaries to be "a young cow." For practical purposes heiferhood, which generally may be said to be a somewhat indefinite period lying between calfhood and maturity, may be taken to be the period between about one year old and the production of the first calf. In this period the animal's life is somewhat different in its aspects, alike from that which precedes and that which follows. Soon after it is a year old the animal is treated with a view to the approach of the time when she shall be bred; as when once she has assumed the duties of motherhood, though not yet in most cases mature, or to be fully mature for two years or more, she is fairly become a cow. The aim in life of the heifer, then, is reproduction of her kind, and the treatment she is to meet with must always have this idea in view. To make life one unvarying round is, therefore, the great object. Monotony is no wearing thing in an animal's life story; on the contrary, when made up of unvarying comfort and plenty, and a strict avoidance of every disturbing element, it is the ideal life for the dumb brute; the *summum bonum* of the purely physical existence. This is no easy thing to attain. Men are not machines, neither are cattle. You cannot set a man, as you can a wheat drill, so that he will give out just so much, no more, no less, throughout the year; nor can you regulate the stock to eat just one amount daily, or to be contented and thrifty on a single kind of food. We must deal with them as individuals; we must look constantly to see that each has enough without having too much. That the heifer maintains good flesh and good health; that she does not grow too fat in summer nor too lean in winter, or at any other time of year. That, in short, plenty and scarcity on the farm do not rotate; and if they do in the fields—for bad seasons will come—that they do not in the feed-box. It is one of the most frequently repeated charges of the many made against cattle-breeders, that they do not give this unvarying attention to their stock; that they especially do not provide for them properly in the late winter and early spring. Now it is of the utmost importance that all the stock should have this regular care and attention, but it seems to me especially necessary for the heifers. They are still as much in a formative state as in calfhood. Their possibilities are half developed and their promise may be checked and made to come to naught by neglect or abuse at this time more than at almost any other period of their lives. Their growth must be kept up by abundant feeding, and the time for breeding them must be determined by their development with a care which shall studiously consider the danger on the one hand of breeding so early as to check and impair the physical development, or so late as to permit the possible supervening of some trouble which shall make them shy in breeding. Very thin and very fat heifers are alike undesirable for breeding purposes. Very thin animals lack vitality and demand too large a part of all the food they get to insure a proper supply of it going to develop a healthy calf. Very fleshy heifers, on the other hand, are in a large number of cases difficult to get to stand, and fat cows are likely to produce very small calves. What is desired is good condition without running to either extreme. To secure this it is only necessary to deal with each animal as an independent organism, and feed just as much as is found necessary and no more. To feed a number of animals on a general average rule often succeeds, but when it does fail it is often in the most unfortunate way, for it gets the easy feeders too high in flesh and they are hard to reduce, and it lets the poor feeders drop behind and they are hard to bring up.

In regard to the age at which a heifer should be bred much depends on the breed, and still more on the actual maturity of each individual animal. Some of the smaller breeds mature earlier than the others and should be bred earlier. The Jerseys and other Channel Island cattle are good illustrations of this class. The Short-horns may be taken as a mean between these and some of the later maturing breeds. My experience with Short-horn heifers is that they should be bred at about eighteen months old. Certainly it is rarely for their ultimate good to be bred earlier than that age. If the heifers are small or backward in any way it is often advantageous to delay breeding from one to three months later. Much depends on the time of calving in the development attained by an animal. Calves which are dropped in the late fall and early winter can rarely compete at eighteen months old with those calved in the spring. When the equation of one calf's life is made up of two winters and a summer it can hardly be expected to compare favorably with that of another which is made up of two summers and a winter. Hence, full allowances must always be made for such things. In a colder climate, too, maturity is retarded; in a warmer climate it is hastened. I speak for my own latitude and give only an average. It will rarely be found advisable to delay the time of breeding so late as until the heifer is twenty-four months old. Two years old is late enough to be a little risky and more time may be lost by several services being required to get such a heifer to stand, if no more serious evil results. Of course no heifer ought to be pushed into the drains of motherhood till her development is sufficient to warrant it, but few heifers are so backward as not to be quite prepared for such drains by the time they are thirty months old.

Wherever practicable young heifers should be bred to young bulls. Old bulls are in most cases too heavy to be safe, and serious dangers are often incurred by breeding to them. I have had heifers killed by the service of a heavy old bull, and less serious injuries are more common. Of course, in a majority of cases if due care is used such accidents will not occur, but they do occur sometimes despite the utmost foresight, and it is wisest to avoid even such possibilities. Where there is no young bull available and an old one must perforce be used, he should in no case be allowed to serve the heifer more than once. A yearling or two-year-old bull is always greatly to be desired for the first service of young females.

When the heifers are eighteen to twenty-four months old, and safely in calf, all that they require in this latitude is good pasturage in summer—such as our blue grass so richly affords—and, in winter, hay and corn-fodder in addition to the scanty food afforded by the winter fields, fed out of doors in racks, or, in the case of the corn-fodder, fed on the ground by being forked out each morning from a wagon. As no more fodder is fed than the cattle eat up cleanly, and the strong turf of the blue grass makes it possible to feed it in a clean spot, there is no waste from this method. I find such fare ample to keep heifers and dry cows in good condition. Where the winter is severe they may profitably be housed at night, though I do this as little as possible, and where they do not keep in good condition on the above described diet it should be supplemented with such grain as the case demands.

As the time of parturition approaches especial attention is demanded. If the time of the year is late winter or early spring, and the animal shows the lassitude and general weakness of the system so generally incident to this time of year, it is well to fortify the system by a little toning up. For this purpose a little grain fed daily for three to four weeks before calving is the best tonic. It is not desirable to feed anything that is heating. and therefore chopped oats, wheat bran, or middlings, with a little oil-cake or flaxseed, is most desirable. Nature is generally at a low ebb at this period and this course has been found very desirable with mares and other animals as well as cows. If, however, the period falls a little later an exactly opposite danger is to be apprehended. When the new vigor of the spring and early summer is abroad in the land, and the animals are lusty and full-blooded from the abundance of rich pasturage, the blood is often in a feverish condition, and if some cooling anti-febrile remedy is not given at the time of calving, puerperal or milk-fever is very likely to ensue. May and June are the months in which this much-dreaded disease is most likely to attack the cows, and during those months it should be most carefully guarded against. It is most liable to attack those that are in high flesh and that are large milkers, and where these conditions are combined in one animal great care should be given to it to guard against this trouble.

In addition to these general subjects of attention young cows with their first calves are often very restless from the time that the premonitory pains of labor begin to come on. As the moment of calving draws near this often increases to a great extent, and the heifer will lie down and then jump up and run about, and often will bring forth her calf when standing up, always imperiling the calf; and too often killing it.

CALVING.

There is no special difference in the treatment required by heifers and cows at the time of calving except that the former require a little more watching, and as the act of bringing forth her first-born ushers the heifer, as it were, into the fuller life of maturity, the subject to which we have now come may be treated in its broadest relations.

When the cow is about to calve she should be left as entirely alone as is consistent with a general oversight and a readiness to interfere if anything goes wrong. Quietness is the great desideratum. In good weather there is no place so good for this purpose as the pasture where the cow has been accustomed to wander at will. In bad weather she should be put in a capacious box-stall where warmth and quiet can be had. The approach of labor can generally be detected early enough for the herdsman to have his attention called to the cow about to calve, and quietly keeping her in his eye she may be watched from a distance and only approached when there is some sign of distress. A very restless heifer is perhaps better put in the stable at once, where she is more apt to lie down and calve in quiet. In general no interference is desirable unless after long labor it is evident that something is wrong. Malpresentations are the most fertile causes of such protracted labor, and artificial means must in such cases be resorted to. If in reach a veterinary surgeon is always desirable, as few amateurs make successful accoucheurs. Where interference is absolutely necessary it must be resorted to, though few can hope to do more than save the cow till they have acquired some costly practical experience.

As has already been said, heifers sometimes need to have their motherly instinct aroused and the calves often need to be helped at the first suckling. Very few calves will take all their dam's milk for the first few days after birth, and the cow must be well milked twice a day for several days after calving. If this is neglected the bag will become clogged with milk and may spoil. The bag should be well milked out, even if the calf seems to empty it, till it is certain the youngster will take it all and strip the bag well. No one who has had the trouble and worry of a spoiled bag on his hands will need to have the necessity of this impressed upon him.

After calving, the principal thing to be looked after is the removal of the placenta, or afterbirth. A healthy cow will "clean" without any attention, and this is the rule. But perhaps no trouble with cows is more common than the retention of the whole or a part of the afterbirth. If the cow's system is in good order nature will do its work; hence the best remedy for this disease is the preliminary prevention which ensures the cow coming to parturition in good health. Where this fails or is neglected it is too late to dally with medicines, and if the cow does not clean within twenty-four hours after calving the afterbirth must be removed by mechanical means. A longer delay than this is not to be risked, as the womb will close and render the removal difficult or impossible except with great risk. The afterbirth should in no case be left unremoved, as it will almost surely lead to blood-poisoning.

I have already adverted to the danger of milk fever in the early summer time in the case of cows of a full habit and deep milkers. The danger is so general that all cows calving at this time of the year should be given a good dose of some cooling purgative. I find that a drench of from one to two pounds of Epsom salts dissolved in as much water as is necessary, which will be about a quart, administered immediately after calving and repeated in five or six hours if it does not act, is an almost certain preventive. I never omit this, as it is beneficial in all cases and highly necessary in some.

Despite all precautions milk fever will sometimes supervene. In that case the most prompt measures must be adopted, as unless taken in the early stages it is almost certain to be fatal. In such a case call in a veterinarian as quickly as one can be secured, for professional treatment of the most skillful sort will have enough to do to save the cow. Where a veterinarian cannot be had at once, or not at all, I know of no better remedy than that recommended by Dr. A. J. Murray, in his admirable little work on "Cattle and Their Diseases." This is tincture of aconite given in the proportion of twenty-five to thirty drops to a pint of thin gruel every three or four hours, beginning with the earliest premonitions of the disease, till 120 to 130 drops have been taken. In connection with the aconite a pound of Epsom salts, mixed with an equal amount of common salt and one ounce of ginger dissolved in three quarts of water sweetened with molasses, is to be given to open the bowels. In case the purge fails to act it is to be repeated, and when that does not promptly give the desired result injections of warm soap suds are to be given till the bowels are thoroughly evacuated. Broken ice in a cloth bag is applied to the head and friction to the limbs. The aconite is of course a simple febrifuge, and is administered solely for the purpose of allaying the fever. As soon as the fever is broken, therefore, it should be discontinued.

It is a singular fact worthy of note, that heifers with their first calves seem to enjoy entire immunity from puerperal fever. I have never known a single case in my long experience, and am quite confident that they are exempt from it.

COWS.

The cow was certainly never intended to be a non-milk-giving animal. I can never sufficiently deprecate, therefore, the neglect of milking qualities in any breed. Milk production being essential to the maintenance of a breed, it is certainly consistent with its character, however much abundant milk production may tax the system. Everything ought to be done to develop the milking qualities of all breeds of cattle, and a little special attention and the feeding of the most suitable food will be found to greatly improve the flow of milk where it has been neglected. Of course in a state of nature cows only gave a comparatively small quantity of milk, and that only for a relatively short period. The demand upon them was irregular and for just the amount required by the calf, and the calf was weaned as soon as it was able to shift for itself. The experience of every farmer is that it injures the milking qualities of the cow to let the cow and calf run together for a long period. The cow "lets down" only small quantities of milk at a time, and when she is called on for a full milking twice a day fails to properly respond. This is well illustrated on the Western ranges, where the cows are small milkers and go dry very early. There is scarcely one of our improved breeds which has not the milk-producing power developed far beyond the original capacity of the unimproved animal. But this quality varies in the animals of every breed and through a wide extent. Not only so, but careful experiments have proved beyond question that milk production in the individual is subject to atrophy and to development. The same animal's production, both in quantity and quality, is dependent on the treatment it receives. If begun with in early life, too, the amount of development possible is far greater than where there has been neglect till after maturity. If we want beef production we must begin in calfhood; if we want milk production we must begin at, or just prior to, the first period of lactation.

A distinguished man of today, when asked when one should begin with a boy to make a scholar of him, is said to have replied: "You must begin with his grandfather." It was an answer on the lines of the old proverb: "You cannot make a silk purse out of a sow's ear." Both teach, when applied to cattle-breeding, the principle of the force of heredity; the value of improved breeds. We cannot make a prize dairy cow out of a scrub. But even the scrub may be made better as a milker by proper care; may be made better, and may be made to produce a calf better than she otherwise would, transmitting the impulse. It is the same thing as the unequaled "corn-crib cross" in the beef breeds. Of course, where milk is the object *par excellence*, the first thing to be done is to select high-class dairy stock. Now, we are only considering the best means of getting all there is in a given lot of cattle out of them, be they good, bad, or indifferent. Given the cows we want to make them yield as much as possible.

It must be remembered that we cannot make something out of nothing. Axiomatic as is this statement it is not practically believed in by many farmers. The demands upon the food merely to maintain life are great. The waste of the system has to be repaired constantly. This is large enough in warm weather; in the winter, when combustion for the creation of heat is so great, it is much larger. And yet men expect to feed cows little more than enough for bare existence and have them produce large quantities of milk. This is utterly ridiculous as well as impossible. Sometimes the natural tendency of milk production, kept alive by the maternal instinct which the tugging of the calf at the teats creates daily anew, will keep a cow in milk when she is little more than a skeleton, but such production is at the expense of the vital energies and means a shortening of life and reduction of future productiveness. About two-thirds of a food ration is needed to supply the demands of mere continued existence. Unless there is something fed over and above this two-thirds, no production of beef or milk can be looked for. The steer that is fed no more will make no gain in weight; the cow that is fed no more will go dry. The question of the difference in care between a dry and milking cow, especially in winter, is dependent on this consideration. A dry cow must be fed only enough to supply the demands that are represented by keeping her in good condition. The milch cow must have enough over and above this to supply the material for the milk. Milk, the chemists tell us, contains all the elements of the animal body (hence its completeness as a food ration); therefore it can only be made by a ration rich in these elements. The food ration for milk must then be a rich one. What the ration lacks the milk will be deficient in. That one cow can be made to give as rich milk as another may not be possible; but by proper food a cow may be made to give richer milk than when fed on improper food.

There is no better ration for milk than abundant pasturage in old pastures. In new meadows of clover only, or of any one grass, there is not enough variety to ensure a full ration; but as the meadows grow older other grasses spring up to give the needed variety and make the ration complete. Hence in the summer good pasturage and plenty of it is all the cows need. But in the seasons of the year when this is not to be had it must be replaced by an abundance of other food. Not only so; as cold is one of the great drains on the animal system and a great consumer of food, shelter is required so that the greatest possible amount of food shall go to milk production. The capacity of assimilation is only just so great and the amount of food is therefore limited, and economy of resources must be practiced. Not only so, but the physiological effects of cold, especially of the chill caused by a sudden change of weather, are very injurious to milk production. Therefore, while the dry cows may find all they require out of doors with fodder and hay, the milking cows require a warm shelter at night and in exceptionally bad weather, and a good milk ration. Mixed wheat, bran and corn-meal, with nice bright clover and timothy hay and chopped oats, proportioned to the cow's powers of production, is as cheap and serviceable a ration as will readily be found.

Milk, it is well to remember, is a fluid, and can only be produced in large quantities where the consumption of water is great. If the water supply is important in all cases, it is doubly so in that of milking cows. Let it be freely obtainable, clean, pure, and wholesome. If it is to be taken in large quantities at once it is better that it should not be at a very low temperature. It is well settled that cows in milk drink far more than cattle in process of fattening, but the exact relations of the amount of water drunk to the milk given can hardly be said to have been determined as yet. Upon this point, however, Prof. Stewart* cites the report of M. Dancel to the French Academy of Sciences upon some very interesting experiments which he had made. He says: "The experiments were to determine the effect of quan-

* "Feeding Animals," pp. 352 and 353.

tity of water upon quantity and quality of milk. By inducing cows to drink more water the quantity of milk yielded by them can be increased in proportion up to many quarts per day without perceptibly injuring its quality. The amount of milk is proportional to the quantity of water drunk. In experimenting upon cows fed in stall with dry fodder that gave only nine to twelve quarts of milk per day," it was found "that when this dry food was moistened with from eighteen to twenty-three quarts of water daily, their yield was then from twelve to fourteen quarts of milk per day. Besides this water taken with the food, the cows were allowed to drink the same as before, and their thirst was excited by adding a little salt to the fodder. The milk produced under this additional amount of water, on analysis, was pronounced of good quality; and when tested for butter was found satisfactory. A definite amount of water could not be fixed upon for each cow, since the appetite for drink differs widely in different animals. He found by a series of observations that the quantity of water habitually drunk by each cow during twenty-four hours was a criterion to judge of the quantity of milk that she would yield per day. And a cow that does not habitually drink as much as twenty-seven quarts of water daily must be a poor milker, giving only five and a half to seven quarts per day. But all the cows which consumed as much as fifty quarts of water daily were excellent milkers—giving from eighteen to twenty-three quarts of milk daily. He gives a confident opinion that the quantity of water drunk by a cow is an important test of her value as a milker."

These tests, it appears, were made on cows much below the standard of first-rate milkers, and they show that a large part of the water consumed was demanded by the animal system. Cows drinking upward of fifty quarts of water gave only eighteen to twenty-three quarts of milk. It will be readily seen that a much greater amount will be demanded by cows giving from thirty-two to forty quarts daily. For such cows a very large amount of water is required.

In handling milch cows it must be borne in mind that the mere mechanical act of milking has not a little to do with a cow's production. Every drop a cow will give must be taken from her night and morning. A poor milker who half milks the cows will let them go dry very quickly. The calves having had their fill, every cow should be carefully stripped, and the cows that are not suckling calves should be milked out carefully. This should be kept up till within two months to six weeks of the next calving. Of course there is a wide variation in the time that cows will naturally remain, or can be kept, in milk. There are some that can, with difficulty, be kept in milk six months among the "natives," and there are many blooded cows which it is difficult to dry off after ten or eleven months. The effect of systematic and long-continued milking is always to increase the period of lactation, and it should be attended to even when, with a young cow, the milking gives so little as to seem not worth the while. It especially behooves the breeders of Short-horn cattle, so long famous for their milking qualities, to see that these are not neglected and gradually lost.

The time in which a cow will come in heat again is somewhat uncertain. A healthy animal suckling her calf will ordinarily come in in from forty to sixty days after calving. She should be bred at once, as early in the heat as convenient, and then put in a quiet place until the excitation of the period of heat has quite worn away. There is no more fertile cause of failure of conception in healthy animals than the excitement of the animal, either by careless driving, by allowing the cow to remain too long with the bull, or to be served too often, or by permitting other cows to fret her. A single service early in the heat and immediate removal to a quiet place is the desirable practice.

With a vigorous bull, whose energies are not

overtaxed, there is no reason why healthy cows, treated in a sensible way, should not stand at the first service. For various reasons, which are in the main not capable of explanation, many cows miss the first and sometimes several services. If no evidences of ill-health are discernible and the bulling is regular, there is nothing to be done but to return the cow at each heat to the bull, or to some other bull. The latter plan sometimes proves at once successful, showing that the difficulty lay with the bull.

All diseases affecting the generative organs are somewhat insufficiently understood. This is especially true of abortion. Abortions fall into two broad classes: those caused by some local trouble of sporadic origin, and those caused by some epidemic or endemic disease.

The sporadic cases of abortion are generally due to some constitutional disease which reacts upon the fœtal system or to some local affection of the womb. Animals affected with any form of tuberculosis are especially subject to abortions. The highly heritable nature of tuberculosis makes it almost a blessing that this is so, for any means that will check the spread of so dangerous and so insidious a disease deserves welcome. There are many other diseases which lead to a general weakness of the system which will induce abortion. Not only active diseases but a general low condition of the system, such as is brought on by the want of proper food and attention during the winter, and which is likely to show itself in the period of extreme lassitude which marks the passing from winter to spring. The treatment in these cases is, if there are sufficient premonitory symptoms to give an opportunity for preventives, perfect quiet and a general toning up of the system. But this rarely occurs. The symptoms of abortion are generally not sufficiently marked to attract attention till too late to take any steps to prevent its occurrence. Youatt, in his celebrated book on cattle, in many respects the pioneer in this field, says that "the cow is, more than any other animal, subject to abortion," and fixes the usual periods of its occurrence at half the natural period of gestation, seven and eight months. Of these periods, that falling at seven months will in a great proportion of cases yield a living calf. The first four to five months, of course, never does, and the eighth month rarely gives a living calf, though I have known one or two to live.

An abortion is unfortunate as losing the calf, but it is a serious trouble, moreover, often destroying the breeding qualities of the cow. Hence cows which abort must be treated with great care. Sometimes the calf dies before expulsion from the uterus and is fetid when ejected, and the afterbirth comes away slowly and is extremely noisome. Such cases are almost invariably followed by great loss of flesh and general breaking down of health. The coat becomes staring and rough, with the cow dull and feverish at first, and a general decline ensues. She comes in heat quickly and is likely to be very irregular in her bulling. Such cases are often fatal, and if there is any taint in the animal's blood by inheritance the congenital defect is sure to show itself. The only treatment is good fare and general tonics. No attempt to breed the cow should be made for weeks, or till she has regained her normal appearance and regularity of heat. Should she be bred while the uterine trouble is actively present she will in most cases fail to stand, and the disease will be aggravated; and, if she should stand, a second abortion would almost surely follow. Indeed, one of the great evils of abortion is that a cow having once aborted may do so again and again in successive years; generally at the same period. This fact, that the time of a subsequent abortion is apt to be approximately that of the preceding, gives warning and enables the owner to make use of preventives.

Where the calf is born alive—or if dead is yet not offensive, showing that it has only died in the immediate process of expulsion—serious results are neither so likely to occur at the moment nor in the future. Nevertheless, the cow should be carefully attended to, only bred after some time of rest, and then watched with a view to prevent a repetition of the disease. Not infrequently it proves impossible to get a cow which has aborted in calf. More often it is a difficult matter, involving great loss of time, and this sometimes is repeated after each succeeding calving for some years. If a cow thus becomes a shy breeder she loses much time and a great part of her value. If she aborts twice in succession it is ordinarily the part of wisdom to feed her off. It is almost sure that her profitableness is gone, and she may be a source of danger to the herd, for it is by no means certain how far the sporadic and the epidemic or epizootic types of this disease run into each other. Most writers think it at least the part of wisdom to remove the fœtus and the afterbirth far beyond sight and smell of the other cows. Youatt strongly recommends this, for he had great doubt of the disease ever being truly contagious, questioned its epidemic character, and fell back on the far more doubtful and questionable theory that it was caused by the effect of imagination. He says: *"The cow is an animal considerably imaginative and highly irritable during the period of pregnancy.

*"Youatt on Cattle," Ed. Stevens, p. 383.

In abortion, the fœtus is often putrid before it is discharged; and the placenta, * * * as it drops away in fragments, emits a peculiar and most noisome smell. This smell seems to be singularly annoying to the other cows—they sniff at it and then run bellowing about. Some sympathetic influence is exercised on their uterine organs, and in a few days a greater or less number of those that had pastured together likewise abort."

The so-called epizootic type of abortion has evaded many later investigators than Youatt, who, if they have agreed in rejecting his theory of the reaction of the imagination on the uterine system, have agreed in little else. Certain it is that this disease is mysterious in its coming and going, its transmission, and many other circumstances of its occurrence, and where it appears it paralyzes production sometimes for one, more often for several years. Those who have suffered from this scourge seem to think it cheaper to wipe out the herd—stopping the conflagration by burning up its fuel in advance—and after an interval to begin afresh, than to try to fight the unequal battle.

I have known of a case where this disease came suddenly, spread rapidly, and went swiftly; of another where it developed gradually, spread slowly but widely, and was only gotten rid of by the destruction of the herd after some years.

It has been attributed to ergot. While ergot, no doubt, does at times cause abortion, this disease has shown itself where ergot was certainly not the cause. It has been thought that the bull was the active agent, but a single bull has been used steadily in two herds, one affected and the other healthy. We can only say it is a mystery.

I wish to accentuate before passing from this subject the high value I set upon the prompt and complete removal of the placenta in all cases of abortion. I have rarely known a cow to suffer seriously in health where this has been done efficiently. In almost every instance it alone seems to give rise to later stages of irritation and inflammation, and with it once out of the way the cow will quickly regain her usual health. If the afterbirth is not removed, like any other foreign animal substance it will decay and induce blood-poisoning, which if not fatal is sure to induce a tedious and troublesome illness, slowly recovered from and often bringing on secondary complaints destructive to the animal's usefulness.

BULLS.

When the bull calves are weaned they require the same treatment which has already been recommended for the heifers and should be kept by themselves, quite apart from the females of the herd. The first crisis in the young bull's life comes when he is between nine and twelve months old. He is then passing from a calf into a bull and change is sure to make him restless and inclined to charge about, and if any cows or heifers are pastured near, especially if they are allowed to run out when in heat, the youngster will worry off all his flesh and get himself thoroughly out of condition. Let him be well secluded, then, given a quiet grass lot and abundant food and pushed along well in his growth, without overfeeding. During this period the young bulls are apt to get uneven and ragged. This is because they are passing from the round, plump, comparatively formless period of calves, and settling down into the well-fixed character of the mature animal. Not a few seem to go through what may perhaps be termed a progressive development. That is, some parts of the body seem to outgrow others, getting their final form first, the others developing more slowly. This often makes a calf of this age more faulty than at any time in his life before or after. There is no reason to despair of the calf of which this is true; good care and time will even up his form. It is often surprising how a good calf will go to pieces at this time and then recover and grow out into all and more than he promised to be. This is not a phenomenon confined to the *genus bos*. It is true of all young males in the period of transition to maturity.

A well-grown yearling bull is capable of performing light service, and it is very desirable to have such an one to breed to yearling heifers. He should of course be used with great caution, very infrequently and on very few cows for the first year. Fifteen or twenty are quite enough for him his first year, and rather more than half of the work had better fall in the second half of the year. As he grows older the number may be steadily and gradually increased, until at five years old, if he is a strong and vigorous animal, he ought to be capable of covering a hundred cows with the certainty of getting a calf in nearly every instance. Of course no bull gets so high a proportion of calves. There are many disturbing causes quite apart from any want of vigor on his part. The chief of these are disease or other causes affecting the females solely. Still a hundred cows is hard service, even for an exceptionally vigorous bull, and he must be well cared for and fed an abundance of strength-supplying food if he is to be expected to be a sure and regular breeder. Let me strongly emphasize the necessity of abundant out-of-door life and exercise for the stock bull. Too much stabling is unnatural and highly enervating, and robs all males of their highest vigor. The close confinement of a stable is likely to be a strain on the general system too, affecting the temper and the nervous organism; and those that are thus kept are often cross-tempered and given to chafing and fretting, and in the end are very likely to become actively vicious. Give the bull a free, open pasture lot, sheltered from the cold winds in the winter days, from the direct rays of the sun in the summer, and let him have at least twelve hours' quiet rumination there in every twenty-four. A young bull, if inclined to be restless in his lot and seemingly at a loss for companionship, may often be better off for a few bull calves in the same enclosure. An old bull showing a like disposition is often made quiet by being allowed to run at least a part of the year with the dry cows. The freedom and the exercise he *must have* or he will lose his potency early; the companionship is not so necessary.

Again, no bull can do heavy service well on pasturage alone, be it ever so good. There is no better food ration than the best pasturage, and it meets the requirements of animals under ordinary conditions most admirably; but a bull doing full service the year round is not living under ordinary conditions and he needs a more condensed ration, one which will give a greater amount of nutritive food for the same bulk.

The pasturage should be supplemented by a liberal allowance—as much as the bull will eat up cleanly in most cases, unless actual experience shows that he inclines to become too fat on such a ration—of cut oats and chopped hay, and a good feed of wheat bran and corn, shelled and crushed if possible. This is necessary to keep up the lusty state of body which is so essential to sexual vigor. Of course this is very different from the course recommended in general with cows, and it deserves special notice. A great many breeders allow their stock bull to run out with their cows, and especially with their dry cows. The result of this is that they get only such food as the cows get. Now, while there is no need of anything more than pasturage, or pasturage and hay and corn-fodder for dry cows, a bull cannot do heavy service on such a ration. Every breeder who has pursued such a course has surely noticed that, while the cows keep in excellent condition, the bull is almost always in low flesh, and not infrequently excessively thin. Where the bull is kept in the pasture with all the cows the milking cows will be housed and fed, and the bull often left out and without feed in the winter. The tax on the bull at the same time is, in its way, quite as great as, even greater than, that upon the system of a cow in milk and in calf. He must be fed to meet this tax; fed, and fed liberally.

How necessary this is may be illustrated by the ordinary treatment which a stallion making a heavy season requires and always receives. No one would expect a horse to do heavy service in the stud on pasturage, however good. On the contrary, the stallion is carefully housed and fed on the most invigorating food, given a regular quantum of exercise, and in most cases used only at certain hours of the day. Why a high-bred bull should not receive the same care cannot be explained. In just the degree of approximation to such care the actual treatment is, in that degree will the excellence of results be. A breeding bull returns in his calves full measure for the care given him, and enough strengthening food must always be fed him to render him lusty and vigorous.

Now this does not mean that the bull is to be overfed. A thin-fleshed bull, running out of doors all the year, is certain to be a surer and better breeder than an over-stabled, overfed one. Obesity leads to lazy, sluggish temper, and a general decay of bodily vigor. Nature abhors extremes. The *via media* is always the wise way. There is no sense in shying at the ditch on one side only to back into that on the other. What is wanted is a bull that is in good condition; that will at the same time go eagerly to the feed trough and eat up his feed quickly and entirely; that will serve a cow promptly and without delay; that, in short, is active, wide awake, and in high health.

In speaking of over-feeding the question of feeding for the show-ring naturally suggests itself. Can a bull be fed, trained and exhibited without impairing his procreative powers? In general it may be safely said that there is great danger in so doing. While a risk is always involved, there is no certainty of doing injury, and to many the object in view will justify the risk. A bull calf, even a yearling bull, may be put in show-yard condition without any serious risk under ordinary circumstances. They will stand a high state of flesh, especially if not cut off from their regular exercise, which would injure maturer animals. On the other hand, few bulls can stand five years of systematic training for the show-ring without loss of vigor. It is a highly unnatural life. The whole fabric of the body is surcharged with an undue amount of fatty matter; the blood is made hot and feverish; the frame soft and lacking in muscle; the internal organs clogged with outside fat; and the whole animal smothered, as it were; every organ impeded in its action by the animal's own flesh. If the animal by nature has a tendency to fat this will be abnormally developed and fatty degeneration of one organ or another will follow. In the bull, as in the cow, the organs of procreation seem to suffer first. Some animals of great vigor stand the strain. They are in most cases animals of a natural and inherited tendency to high flesh; animals which take on a show-yard form with great ease and rapidity, and without the great strain that most animals have to be subjected to. They can be kept in ordinary flesh till within a few weeks of the exhibition season and then put in a sufficiently good state. By taking them out of the breeding establishment for the time, and letting them have a further rest from service after the season's fairs are over, they will show in many cases few or no evil effects. It is rare that such animals are found. It is because there are some such that the standard in the fair-ring is based on what is obesity for most animals. And so long as these things are so the few will set the example and the rest will simulate a virtue which they do not possess. I have shown with great success, and without any real injury, several of my best breeding bulls from calfhood or yearlings to maturity. Among these were such celebrated bulls as Muscatoon, Chilton, Loudon Duke, and Baron Butterfly. But no one of these bulls was ever overdone. They took on flesh with great ease and rapidity, and were always in sufficiently high flesh to content those who could not see excellence apart from high flesh, and their native excellence was hard to be passed over. But it is hard to win with a thin bull, however good. His want of flesh may be to the penetrating eye of an expert but the result of ordinary feeding and heavy work; but the less experienced will inevitably think that he is thin because corn and oats, and oil-cake, etc., etc., etc., *ad infinitum*, could not make him a mountain of flesh, such as many of his competitors are sure to be. As a practical question I should meet this matter of overfeeding by strong advice against subjecting a valuable animal to it. At the same time I do not advise against the exhibition of really first-class animals, nor exhibiting them in good condition. Good judges will see their merit and they will win despite ignorance and the prevailing faults of our show-rings. Such triumphs are the kind that tell in the way of solid reputation, and they are the greatest educators. The uninformed looker-on usually thinks the largest bull is going to win, no matter how coarse he may be, no matter how patchy and badly disposed the flesh may be upon his huge ungainly carcass. If such an one does win it is thought all right; no comment is excited, no inquiry awakened. If, on the other hand, a compact, level, well-formed, but comparatively low-fleshed bull wins, there is at once a question made and his merits are canvassed, generally to the advantage of all lookers-on, who come to understand that the closest approximation to the huge proportions of the elephant is not the highest standard of excellence for a bull of a beef breed of cattle.

In the position which I have here taken I am not simply expressing the results of my own experience, nor yet that of many fellow-breeders and exhibitors of cattle, but I am glad to know that the experiments and investigations of the most eminent theorists, such as Prof. Henry* of the Wisconsin Agricultural Experiment Station, entirely coincide with the views above given as to the danger of and the injuries consequent upon the overfeeding of breeding animals.

In using the bull it is well to remember that his powers are not unlimited, and that in order to secure the best results his faculties must be conserved. In the first place he must not be allowed to cover too many cows. Such a practice brings its own punishment; many of the cows failing to stand, and the calves begotten in many cases failing to reach the standard shown by the get of the same bull when not overworked. If a bull is desired to be highly prepotent he must be given very light work. In order to husband his powers let him first, as already recommended on other grounds, be kept alone, or at most with the dry cows. Secondly, let the cows be taken to his lot to be

*See papers in the *Breeder's Gazette* for 1887.

bred, and never let him serve a cow but once at a single heat. The cow after having been served should be taken away at once, completely out of the neighborhood of the bull. At first he will try to follow her, but he will soon learn to understand the procedure, and having served the cow will walk off and make no effort to follow her. Such a training I esteem of the greatest value. There is no fret, no nervous running about, no bawling after the cow; and this is no less for the good of the bull than, as we have already seen, it is for the cow. Sometimes a cow that has given trouble about standing may be turned in and allowed to run with the bull for several hours, when he will serve her several times. This sometimes leads to a shy breeder being got with calf, but it is a bad, rather than a good, plan for a regular breeding cow, and is not desirable for the bull. It should be a rare exception, and used as a forlorn hope only.

In conclusion let me urge, what has been touched on already above, namely, the reaction on the bull's temper and disposition of his treatment. Handle a bull gently and kindly from the time he is calved until he attains to maturity and grows into old age, and there will be very little to complain of in his temper. If never aroused, the temper of most animals, especially if of a heavy bodily habit, is kindly.

The bulls of the smaller breeds are far more likely to be vicious than those of the large beef breeds. I have never bred or raised a vicious bull in all my life-long experience. It is kindly, watchful, firm handling that is needed, without roughness or abuse. When such care is given the bull will in almost every case be docile and perfectly easy of control.

FEEDING METHODS.

It is not my purpose in this chapter to enter into any exhaustive discussion of the question of cattle feeding. Such a discussion would necessarily occupy a disproportionately large amount of space and would be out of keeping with the general plan of this work. I shall only undertake to outline what has proved in my experience the most practical method of feeding breeding cattle, and to seek to show that there is a middle line between the wasteful old-fashioned methods and the highly specialized, and often in actual application very expensive, methods of the theorists.

I have no quarrel with the theorists. They are the guides of all practical men. That they are often impractical themselves is no reflection on their work. It is the experience of all time that a man is moulded by his pursuits. The student of matter is blinded by the one subject held close to his eyes, and forgets that there is a great world beyond of far different phenomena, and he is led, step by step, into a materialistic belief which reckons on no world but that of matter. He who studies mental phenomena, and the phenomena of soul and spirit, loses his hold on matter and becomes an idealist. He who deals with pure theory, in whatever sphere, views things only in the abstract, and forgets the trammels of daily life. But the results of the theorist's labors are only the more broadly true that they are worked out in connection with abstract truth. The more completely any phenomena, or set of phenomena, can be separated from the concrete cases in which they occur, the more catholic will the cause underlying them be. When the law is once ascertained the man of practical affairs steps in, takes the general truth and applies it to the various needs of the world of action.

Thus, the early experiments in feeding rations appeared visionary and absurd to many practical men. As time went on the essential truth in the theories became more and more apparent, and through the intervention of men at once learned and trained in applying theory to practice the results of the scientific tests have been brought nearer and nearer to the feeder.

I have more to complain of in the old happy-go-lucky way of feeding stock. The theory that "the method my father and grandfather followed is good enough for me," is one of the worst ever formulated. It in almost every case indicates that the inherited method was an unwise and careless one. Had it been otherwise the son and grandson would have been educated by it up to a progressive spirit, for he who is first is always inspirited to maintain his preeminence. Traditions of this sort are usually harbored by those whose fences are rotten, whose weeds are uncut, whose cattle are half-starved in the winter and half-cared for all the year round. We look on the fancy farm of the man who is a follower of pure theory, and then on the run-down farm of "the son of his fathers," and wonder which reaps the least profit. What we want to learn is, what the theoretical scientist has to teach us, and then apply it in a practical, common-sense way. Thus, and thus only, can cattle be fed profitably in this day, when the farmer needs to save every cent he possibly can; save, too, not by hoarding, but by using the most progressive methods and making two profits where formerly only one was made. Let us glance, then, very briefly at the salient facts which science has to teach us in regard to feeding methods before looking at the way the practical feeder deals with the problems which confront him daily

All animal bodies, from the simplest to the most complex, consist chiefly of the four elements of oxygen, hydrogen, carbon and nitrogen. These elements play an equal part in the composition of plants. That part of the bodies of animals and plants which is combustible is made up of these four elements; that which is incombustible—which in chemical analysis forms what is called "ash"—is made up of a variety of elements, among which may be enumerated: sulphur, phosphorus, potassium, sodium, iron, chlorine, magnesium, bromine and iodine. These incombustible elements vary greatly in quantity in different parts of the animal organism, and as a whole constitute but a small part of the body.

The largest constituent of animal bodies is water, which is made up of oxygen and hydrogen in the proportion of two parts of hydrogen to one of oxygen. The per cent of water in any given animal varies with the individual; and also in the individual according as it is fat or lean, a very fat animal containing a smaller proportion of water than a lean one. The amount of water ranges from about thirty-five to seventy per cent. The remainder of the body consists of solid matter of various sorts.

Now life is simply a burning up of the animal body. Oxygen is taken in through the lungs, is carried by the blood throughout the system, and combines with other elements in the body just as the materials of a candle do when it is burned. Constant supplies must be kept up, therefore, to replace the parts burned up or the animal will be consumed; that is, will die of starvation. Not only must the supplies be kept up, but they must be of the character of the parts consumed, and in a form such that the organism will assimilate them. The body may be said to be made up of the blood, muscle, fat, bones, skin, hair, horns, etc.; and each of these has its own particular composition. Thus the blood is made up of nearly eighty per cent of water and a little more than twenty per cent of solids, of which nearly one per cent is ash (chloride of sodium and phosphates of magnesium, soda and lime), and the remainder is a richly nitrogenous matter—very like the white of eggs—with a little fat and sugar. The bones, on the other hand, have about two-thirds of inorganic matter in their constituents, being rich in phosphates of lime and magnesia, in carbonate of lime, in potash and common salt (chloride of sodium). It is necessary for an accurate theoretical determination of the problems of feeding that all the parts of the body should be carefully analyzed and an accurate determination reached as to the relative demand made upon the feeder for food of the various kinds.

Now it is not necessary when this is determined to go to work and get all these elements separately and form a mixture as a physician might compound a prescription and administer the food in such a way. On the contrary, even when the ingredients are actually present they must be in a form adapted to the animal's internal economy. Nature has not only ordained the composition of the food, but its form. It was once thought that animals had the power of transforming materials from their simple elemental form to a more complex state; of preparing food for their own supply by modifying it to suit their needs. But this view is no longer commonly accepted. It is the part of plants to convert the mineral matter of the soil and air into the form needed by animal bodies, and animals can only make use of it when so converted. Hence it would follow that the composition of animals and plants is nearly the same so far as component elements go. And this is quite true. The food of plants consists mainly of water (oxygen and hydrogen), carbonic acid (carbon and oxygen), and ammonia (hydrogen and nitrogen). These, as we have seen, are the principal elements of animal bodies. Not only is this so, but plants also have incombustible elements in their composition, and these are similar to those found in animal bodies. Hence it follows that nature has prepared in plants just the complex food that such animals as the ruminants—to which class the ox belongs—demand. Our task is not a hard one in general, then. Follow nature; feed the stock as nearly as possible as they fed themselves in a state of nature. So true is this that we find the only single substance which affords what the scientist terms a complete ration—that is to say, affords all the elements needed by the animal in the best proportions—is milk. But we find that in any pasture in which a variety of grasses grow, as in ordinary cases is sure to occur, these grasses as a whole afford a complete ration. A little study of the animal's habits will show that instinct has taught it to seek a variety of foods as if for this very purpose of making one supply what the other lacked; of making one supplement the other. A mixed ration of the ordinary products of a farm always offers, therefore, an admirable ration. But nature tends to be lavish; science aims to be economical. The scientist who laboriously works out the exact ration demanded by a two-year-old steer weighing thirteen hundred pounds, in order to gain one and a half pounds per day for six months, will perhaps find when he has finished his task that it is as it stands worthless to the feeder, because he has taken a world-wide field in his calculations of food supplies while the former has only three or four at his command. But the general rule having been reached, the analysis of various foods made, substitutions and variations in the tables can be made at any time without trouble. The first tables puzzled and amused the farmers, but now a table that will work well in practice can readily be made out on the basis of the early German experiments.

The first thing the feeder wants to get settled is what food supplies has he to draw from. Then he can build up on that basis. The breeder needs nothing so much as good permanent pastures. As has already been said, such pastures yield such a variety of grasses as to furnish a complete and most excellent ration. The pasture is the backbone of cattle-breeding. No effort is too great to get the pasture ready for the cattle in the earliest days of spring, or to prolong in the autumn the time during which it yields good grass. The ration afforded by pasturage is not one calculated to make animals very fat. It is well-balanced, tending to make growth and lean meat, rather than fat. In such cases, as fattening is the prime object, an addition must be made of some food rich in fat-making qualities. In such a case the scientist is ready with a suggestion. He will point out that some parts of some plants are digestible and others indigestible, that the nutrition derived from one plant will be greater than that derived from another on this account simply, aside from the question of composition. Thus rye straw is a poor food compared with wheat straw—though chemically very nearly the same—because the latter is more digestible. When this additional factor is brought in the question is fairly open and the things to be determined are, first: The kind of food that is needed to make the kind of growth demanded; second, the kind of plant or grain which offers that food; and third, the digestibility, or, as it is called, the nutritive ratio of the given plant. The cereal grains, the seeds—such as linseed, cottonseed, etc.—rich in oils are specially valuable for pressing forward flesh-making, because they are composed of the elements used in that process.

An animal may pine and die for want of food when heavily fed, if the food is not of the right character. Thus sugar is highly nutritious, but an animal could not subsist upon it for any extended period. What is mainly needed are those elements rich in nitrogen, called in general albuminoids, whose function is muscle-making. All the grains are rich in these materials. After them come certain nutrients, non-nitrogenous in their composition, and called carbo-hydrates because they are made up of carbon and hydrogen and oxygen—and the latter two elements in such proportion as to form water. The stalks of plants, etc., largely consist of these non-nitrogenous matters.

So well has nature distributed these food supplies that often a single plant furnishes an entirely sufficient ration. Thus corn and corn-fodder form a well-recommended ration for feeding fat cattle. The grain and straw of wheat also offer a good ration. There is scarcely any better combination for breeding-cattle than one formed of clover hay, cut oats, and wheat-bran or corn-meal.

It is evident, therefore, that it is not necessary to concoct some elaborate mixture of a great variety of food stuffs in order to get a good ration. Indeed one of the things which scientific investigation has clearly shown is that a little variety in feeding is all that is needed.

What the practical farmer wants is the cheapest ration which is also a good ration. The best way to get at this is generally to consider what is the cheapest food in the section in which we live each year and make that the basis. If wheat is very low bran will probably be one of the cheapest substances we can use. Corn may be still cheaper. The usual fluctuations in the markets may drive us from one food to another, but it will pay to change if many head are to be fed through the winter. Wheat bran, clover hay, and cut oats is one of the best combinations I have ever tried, and for a little increase of flesh production a small addition of linseed-oil cake is very good. Under ordinary circumstances I do not believe that cooked and steamed food is desirable, particularly from an economic point of view. Corn is more heating than wheat bran, but its excellence as a cattle food cannot be denied. For young animals it is best fed as meal; for older animals roughly crushed. The rationale of this is obvious. The smooth, flinty, outer coatings of the grain do not offer a ready access to the gastric juices and a large part of the grain passes out into the draught unaffected by the digestive processes. A great economy is, therefore, effected by feeding crushed corn. Of course in all cases the hay or straw should be fed with the grain. The digestive processes of all ruminants require an abundance of "roughness" for healthy action.

There is no room for dogmatism in the matter of foods. All sorts of grains roots, forage plants, etc., have their claims, and it is largely a question of locality, and what can be cheaply and advantageously grown in any given place. I find no single thing more useful in feeding than sorghum. It has the greatest fattening qualities, is eaten greedily, increases to a marvelous degree the flow of milk, and from the end of August to the first of December it is one of my chief resources. What sorghum is to me, roots are in the farm economy of Canada. They cannot raise sorghum to advantage; we cannot raise roots. Each latitude must adapt itself to its climatic and other conditions.

The feeding of such green food on pasture-land in the summer is an old custom and one which has enjoyed a deserved popularity. There are drawbacks to this system of soiling, but these drawbacks are chiefly found where soiling is carried to a great extreme and made the exclusive method of feeding. Partial soiling in conjunction with good grazing is one of the best methods ever used to put stock in fine condition. Few feeders of show cattle can be found who have not been accustomed to resort to cut ears of green corn, corn-fodder, sorghum, or some similar crop. General soiling on rye, clover, timothy, millet, peas, etc., etc., has not been used to any great extent in this country outside of city dairies or small farms where grass is too scarce to carry the stock. There is no doubt that soiling can be practiced very effectively and economically where land is dear. Its greatest drawback is the cost of labor necessary to keep a crop always in season.

The great problem has been how to procure green food in winter. Dairy cattle especially require such a diet, and the milk flow suffers for lack of it. The silo has been invented as a solution of this problem with very considerable success. The methods now in use took their rise in the experiments of M. Gaffart, in France, and he showed that soiling plants could be preserved through weeks and months in a green state in a compact form and fed with great advantage. The juices of the plants undergo a fermentation which does not impair their usefulness if properly conducted; but it is necessary that the silo should be so constructed as to exclude all air, as the hermetic sealing of the silo is an essential condition of this fermentation taking place without souring. New appliances are making the construction of silos more and more easy and satisfactory, and the time is probably not far off when the use of ensilage will be quite common. There is certainly immense scope for the development of such a system. The difficulties are of course very real and very patent. The cost of the silo is considerable, and in most sections of the country the making of silage has not passed beyond the stage of experiment. The cost of labor, too, tells heavily in these days of slow returns and small profits. But greater than any other difficulty is the general want of practical knowledge which has caused many who have made the experiment to fail, and discouraged others who would otherwise have been glad to make the attempt. This will, no doubt, give way before greater experience, and in a dozen years or more ensilage is likely to play an important part in our farm economy.

Let me now give an average case taken

chiefly from Prof. Stewart's valuable work on "Feeding Animals," and by him drawn mainly from the experiments of Prof. Johnson and Dr. Wolff. He takes as a ration for an average milch cow, estimated for 1,000 pounds live weight, a combination that will contain twenty-four pounds of dry organic substance. This ration should contain of digestible nutrients: albuminoids, two and five-tenths pounds (2.5 lbs.); carbo-hydrates, twelve and five-tenths pounds (12.5 lbs.); fat, four-tenths of a pound (0.4); making a total of fifteen and four-tenths (15.4) pounds in the whole ration of twenty-four pounds. The actual weight of the ration will of course be considerably in excess of this owing to the water, which is not calculated. Thus to get twenty-four pounds of dry matter in young clover hay about twenty-five per cent would have to be added, making say thirty pounds. In such food as mangolds, brewers' grain, etc., a much larger allowance must be made for water, amounting to from seventy-five to as much as eighty-five per cent. The richest and best meadow hay approximates closely the theoretical standard, as may be seen by the following table of analysis (estimated on basis of 1,000 lbs. live weight):

	Total organic dry matter.	*Albuminoids.*	*Carbo-hydrates.*	*Fat.*	*Total nutrients.*
Standard................	24.0	2.5	12.5	0.40	15.40
30 lbs. meadow hay	23.2	2.49	12.75	0.42	15.66

Good rations, fitted to ordinary use, may be readily compounded on the basis of this standard, of which the following are examples:

TABLE I.

	Dry organic substance	*Digestible albuminoids*	*Carbohydrates.*	*Fat.*
12 lbs. average meadow hay	9.5	0.65	4.92	0.12
6 lbs. oat straw	4.9	0.08	2.40	0.04
20 lbs. mangolds	2.2	0.22	2.00	0.02
25 lbs. brewers' grain	5.6	1.20	2.81	0.30
2 lbs. cotton-seed cake	1.6	0.66	0.35	0.12
65-lb. ration containing	23.8	2.81	12.48	0.60
Standard	24.0	2.50	12.50	0.40

TABLE II.

20 lbs. cured corn-fodder	13.7	0.64	8.68	0.20
5 lbs. rye straw	4.1	0.04	1.82	0.02
6 lbs. malt sprouts	5.0	1.25	2.62	0.05
2 lbs. cotton-seed meal	1.6	0.66	0.35	0.12
33-lb. ration containing	24.4	2.59	13.47	0.39
Standard	24.0	2.50	12.50	0.40

TABLE III.

15 lbs. corn-fodder	12.1	0.16	5.55	0.04
5 lbs. bran	4.1	0.59	2.21	0.15
5 lbs. malt sprouts	4.1	1.04	2.19	0.08
3 lbs. corn-meal	2.5	0.25	1.82	0.14
2 lbs. cotton-seed meal	1.6	0.66	0.35	0.12
30-lb. ration containing	24.4	2.70	12.12	0.53
Standard	24.0	2.50	12.50	0.40

The simplest tables, containing only bran or crushed corn, with hay and chopped oats, are, in my judgment, the best for the practical farmer, and may be readily calculated. But while the tables of the scientific investigator are the touchstones to try our work by, even those who prepare them admit that they are only approximate. The personal equation is constantly coming in to cause slight variations, which must be met by constant and unflagging watchfulness on the part of the feeder. Combinations of good hays, clover, timothy, meadow fescue, mixed meadow hay, etc., with chopped oats, wheat bran, or middlings, corn in meal or crushed, never fail, if judiciously mixed, to give excellent results. These are the staples of good feeding. Good results may be obtained from soiling and the use of oil-cakes and meals in special cases, but I am strongly of the opinion that year in and year out the simplest diet is the best. The general use of all condimental foods I am especially inclined to condemn. They are not needed with sound, healthful breeding-cattle. Where they are needed the best way to meet the case is by sending the beast to the block. Cattle which require to be kept up by stimulants are not fit to breed from, and the sooner they cease to perpetuate their feeble race the better.

Of course, where special circumstances intervene, special means must be resorted to. Extraordinary show-yard condition can only be attained by resorting to special methods of feeding. Here, no doubt, all the appliances of forcing may be used with propriety, provided it be first decided that the end in view justifies the extraordinary strain on the animals' systems. But in general all that is really to be sought is to keep the stock in good condition, and hence all specially stimulating, heating, and fat-producing food should be avoided so far as possible.

The great problems of feeding are connected with the fattening of market cattle, and, interesting as they are, lie beyond the proper purview of this work. The fat-stock shows have thrown a flood of light on these matters, and it is perhaps not too much to hope that the day is not far distant when more systematized and scientific, and consequently more economical, methods of feeding will generally prevail. What the practical breeder most needs to learn as to feeding may be summed up in two words: liberality and self-restraint. No man can ever afford to stint his stock, nor yet to overfeed them. Our cattle must have a liberal amount of good, wholesome food, fed with regularity. They want, on the other hand, just as little pampering as possible. Liberality does not mean wastefulness. Thorough-paced economy is not only consistent with it, it is even its twin virtue. Nor yet does self-restraint mean niggardliness. It is no doubt true that the middle road is ill-defined. It is quite as true that it is the best road. It takes patient study, watchfulness and work to keep to it. But then cattle-feeding is a practical man's occupation, not a holiday recreation.

INDEX.

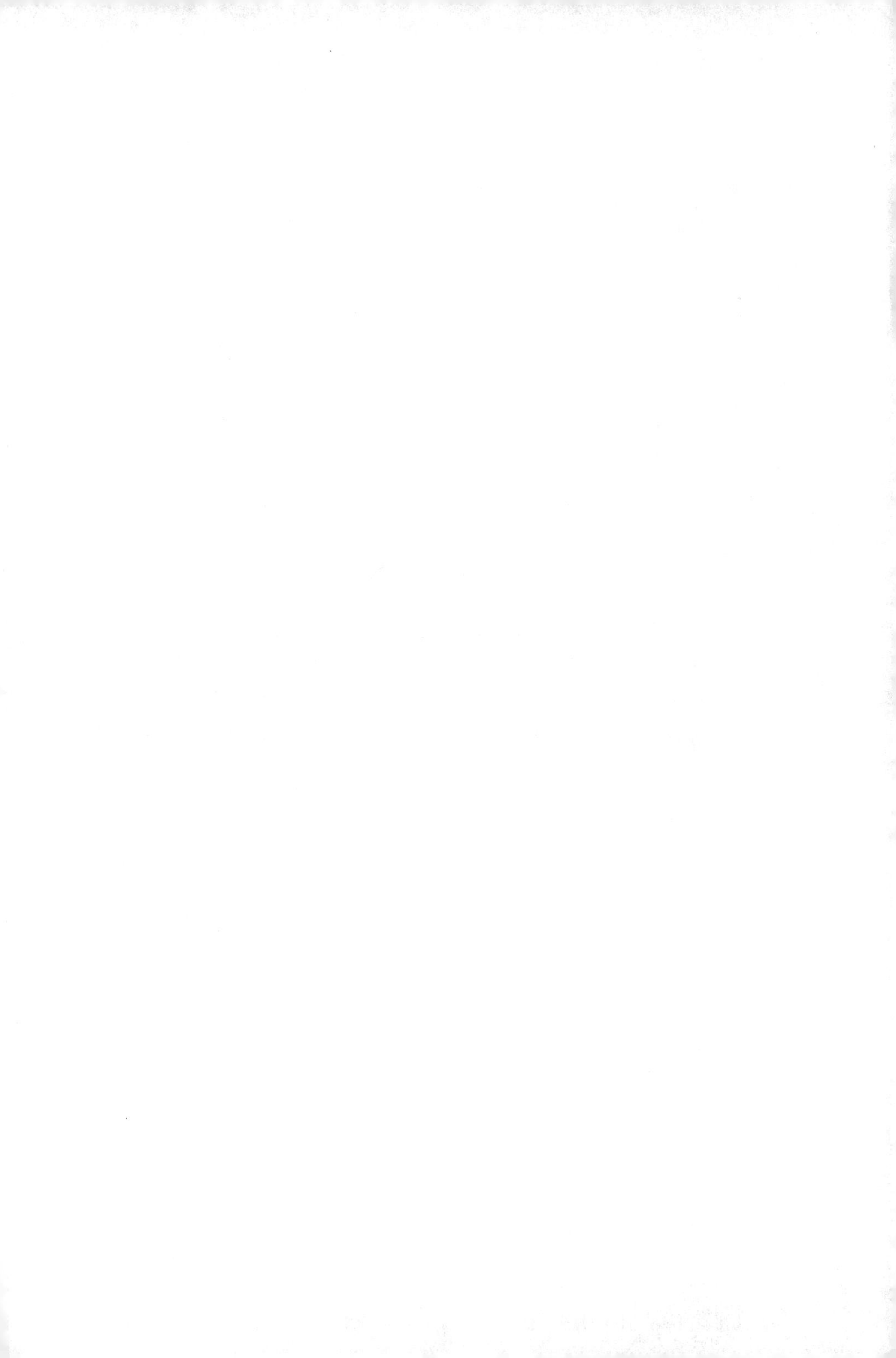

www.ingramcontent.com/pod-product-compliance
Lightning Source LLC
Chambersburg PA
CBHW030859270326
41929CB00008B/498
* 9 7 8 3 3 3 7 1 4 3 5 4 1 *